KU-756-335

You've Got It In You:

A Positive Guide to Breastfeeding

Emma Pickett

Copyright © 2016 Emma Pickett

The moral right of the author has been asserted.

Apart from any fair dealing for the purposes of research or private study,
or criticism or review, as permitted under the Copyright, Designs and Patents
Act 1988, this publication may only be reproduced, stored or transmitted, in
any form or by any means, with the prior permission in writing of the
publishers, or in the case of reprographic reproduction in accordance with
the terms of licences issued by the Copyright Licensing Agency. Enquiries
concerning reproduction outside those terms should be sent to the publishers.

Matador
9 Priory Business Park,
Wistow Road, Kibworth Beauchamp,
Leicestershire. LE8 0RX
Tel: 0116 279 2299
Email: books@troubador.co.uk
Web: www.troubador.co.uk/matador
Twitter: @matadorbooks

ISBN 978 1784624 910

British Library Cataloguing in Publication Data.
A catalogue record for this book is available from the British Library.

Printed and bound in the UK by TJ Books Limited, Padstow, Cornwall
Typeset in 11pt Aldine401 BT by Troubador Publishing Ltd, Leicester, UK

Matador is an imprint of Troubador Publishing Ltd

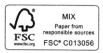

MIX
Paper from
responsible sources
FSC® C013056

You've Got It In You:
A Positive Guide to Breastfeeding

NEWHAM LIBRARIES

90800101148783

Contents

Author's Note

The title – *You've Got it in You* – obviously refers to two things. You've got the breastmilk actually physically literally IN you. Even if you don't exclusively breastfeed for whatever reason, even if you have tiny amounts of glandular tissue and have had some breast surgery, you will produce some milk. Every millilitre counts.

And you've got it in you. You have the determination and commitment to give breastfeeding the best chance possible. When breastfeeding doesn't go to plan, it will be your inner strength that keeps you going and hopefully helps you to overcome the hurdles along the way.

And my son, the eldest of my two breastfed children, came up with the title.

Illustrations and front cover design by Estelle Morris http://www.estellemorris.co.uk/

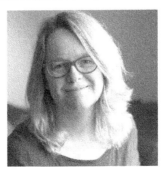

Introduction

Let's remember that for most families throughout history, breastfeeding has been straightforward, normal and easy. It's just what happens after the giving birth bit. It isn't complicated. It isn't scary. It's not something we 'hope' will work and we need to 'give it a go'. Among all the millions and billions of women who have given birth in history, few imagined that for even one moment that it WOULDN'T work. Of course it's going to. Our bodies can make a baby. Why on Earth would the producing milk bit not work? That's a heck of a lot less complicated.

You may be worried about breastfeeding. You may be

Among all the millions and billions of women who have given birth in history, few imagined that for even one moment that it WOULDN'T work – of course it's going to work. Our bodies can make a baby. Why on Earth would the producing milk bit not work? That's a heck of a lot less complicated.

worried that it might not work. This is a common feeling when you live in a society where breastfeeding is often sabotaged by incorrect information, patchy support from a stretched health service and powerful messages from formula companies. But it's not a feeling that is entirely logical. We are mammals. We get our name from the dangly milk-producing bits. It defines us.

I want you to read this book and other books and websites and get informed and I also want to give you a sense of confidence that this is probably going to work if you want it to. It's very likely to. If we positively prepare to breastfeed, our mental state is in a good starting position. I would like you to be as well-prepared as possible. I would like you to breastfeed for as long as you want to and as happily as possible. I want you to feel supported.

I have been a breastfeeding counsellor with the Association of Breastfeeding Mothers (www.abm.me.uk) since 2007 and an IBCLC (International Board Certified Lactation Consultant) since 2011. I have been volunteering on the National Breastfeeding Helpline since it opened in 2008 and have spoken to more than 2000 callers. I have been volunteering at three drop-in groups a week in North London since 2007 and visit new families in their homes and sometimes in hospital. I've seen a lot of tears from people who are struggling to make breastfeeding work.

I've seen a lot more tears from people for whom breastfeeding WAS working but they just didn't know what was normal or how life with a new baby was going to go. Information helps.

The beginning of this book is structured as a timeline. There are things that I would like you to think about when you are pregnant and as each month passes certain issues are likely to crop up. Later on there are some tidbits you may dip into as you go along.

Everyone's experience is different. Everyone's baby is different. Any book that tells you that you MUST breastfeed for X number of minutes should be thrown across the room right now. Or a book that tells you that you can control your baby so that they will want to feed every three hours and if you can't manage that, you're doing something wrong.

There is one universal truth: your baby is a person too. This new little person is coming to share your life and they have their own biological urges and their own needs and they cannot be entirely controlled. Nor should we want to 'control' them. We will fill them with love and they will fill us with love. It might not always feel

I've seen a lot more tears from people for whom breastfeeding WAS working but they just didn't know what was normal or how life with a new baby was going to go.

that magical and at times it will feel incredibly tough. If I tell you that, it doesn't mean I'm not being positive. I am not going to make this sound like a walk in the park in some attempt to convince someone who may be unsure to breastfeed. I want you to be realistically prepared. I want you to understand when things might get hard and how to deal with them. If we know what's normal, it goes a long way to helping us cope with the first few weeks and months.

Some of this new life will be about flexibility and responsiveness and acceptance. If you are used to a world of schedules and decisions and goals, it may be a bit of a shock. Learn about human biology before you think it sounds bit too scary. Babies are the products of millions of years of evolution and we are too, if we can just tap into our instincts and trust them a little bit.

Success comes when we tap into those instincts and when we know when to get help when our instincts aren't answering all of our questions.

Can everyone who wants to breastfeed make it work? No. It may not work out for every single person. Not everyone may be able to exclusively breastfeed due to medical issues. Most of these people can give their baby breastmilk though and I'll talk this through as well. And let's not start this journey by imagining you'll be someone who won't make it.

You're Pregnant

For most women, there is no 'decision' to breastfeed. It seems obvious. It takes a tiny bit of googling to read the research articles on SIDS, allergies, diabetes, obesity, breast cancer, hospitalisation in the first year of life, diarrhoea, respiratory infection, ear infections and so on. However not many women 'decide to' after reading scientific research. It just feels like the right thing to do for many of us. We can see from statistics that starting off breastfeeding is the norm for the current generation of new mums. In England, 74% of mothers initiate breastfeeding after birth. You may be in an area where that figure is a little less or dramatically higher.

Most families want to give it a go. But let's watch our language at this point. Are you thinking: "I'm going to give it a try. It might not happen but might as well try. I'll have formula just in case. I'm not sure it will work out." If you are thinking along those lines, that's a useful sign you need to do more reading and have a better sense of how breastfeeding works. It suggests you don't know many people who have successfully breastfed and haven't been around breastfeeding much. It suggests you may have known more people who struggle and haven't had all the support they wanted.

That applies to many women who live in the UK. Most of us have never seen breastfeeding up close until we have our own baby and we're the ones doing it. We may never have really looked at a nipple in detail before. (Newsflash: the milk comes out of more than one hole!) The only breastfeeding we might have seen was perhaps in a television advert for formula where messages were carefully cultivated. The only women we've seen talking about feeding choices were on bus stop adverts talking about 'moving on from breastfeeding'. We live in a messy culture where we do sort of know breastfeeding is what those breast things are for but we struggle to talk about it. We struggle to do it in front of other people. Breastfeeding support is patchy and many mothers don't get to breastfeed for as long as they want and feel angry and betrayed about their early experiences.

Your job in pregnancy is to get your soldiers lined up and get on the ready line.

74% of women in England start out breastfeeding. By six to eight weeks, how many do you think are still breastfeeding? 60%? Really? That's quite a drop-off rate.

Actually according to Department of Health figures, at the six to eight week check, only 47% of mothers are still doing *any* breastfeeding.

We know from the government's infant feeding survey that many women give up unhappily. Of those who give up in the first two weeks, 90% didn't want to. People give up because they are sore (so lacked support on positioning and attachment). They give up because they feel they don't have enough milk (so often that means they lacked support on positioning and attachment again as a poor latch means less stimulation to your milk supply). Mothers sometimes give up breastfeeding because they simply don't know what normal patterns of baby behaviour look like. They haven't been told what cluster feeding is, or a growth spurt, or how often a baby might feed. They doubt themselves and they doubt what their bodies can do.

Newsflash: the milk comes out of more than one hole!

If you are well-informed, supported by people close to you and supported by people who know about breastfeeding, it is very, very likely you will be in the group who breastfeed for as long as they want to. The group of women who are physically unable to breastfeed is estimated to be between 1-5% of the population. In 1970, breastfeeding rates in Norway were as low as those in Britain today. The country made a concerted effort to change their approach to breastfeeding support. Today 98% of Norwegian women start out breastfeeding, and 90% are still breastfeeding four months later.

Read about breastfeeding. It's really easy to become focused on labour and birth when you are thinking about 'getting ready for baby'. People also end up focusing on buying stuff and choosing names and decorating. It's easy to think, "I'll get to the breastfeeding bit." Especially if you are in the camp already saying, "I'll just be giving it a go." The reality is that women who learn about breastfeeding and inform themselves are far more likely to make breastfeeding work. Not many of us grew up around breastfeeding. There are little girls in the world who see breastfeeding around them all day every day. They absorb the correct body positions and how a baby's mouth gapes and how often auntie seems to be feeding their newborn without even knowing that's what they're doing. They are winding babies and changing breastfed baby poos and practising by holding their dollies as soon as they can hold anything. We miss out on a lot of that. So why would we expect breastfeeding just to happen automatically and instinctively? It is true that breastfeeding is about instinct and natural reflexes and we're built to do it as a species. But that's true of giving birth too and not many people are comfortable to walk into a labour ward without any preparation and without anyone on staff to lend a hand.

Are you a bit scared about how breastfeeding might go? I wonder if that's a positive thing. I think it could be. That suggests this is important to you and that's going to help a lot.

Breastfeeding may be natural but that doesn't mean it's easy for everyone. To start off, there are some useful books out there like "The Womanly Art of Breastfeeding" published by La Leche League. You want evidence-based information from people who are trained in breastfeeding support and experienced. That book you've got on your shelf written by a well-known nanny who has filled 200 pages with guidance on how to care for your newborn? Do you really think she's going to compare to a lactation consultant or a doctor like Jack Newman who focuses on breastfeeding all day long? Will her twenty pages on breastfeeding do the trick? Unlikely. There are popular books out there that contain fundamental misunderstandings about how breasts work and milk supply operates. They wouldn't be allowed to put such errors on a television advertisement. They can just sell them to thousands of new parents every year. You may have bought the well-known baby care book because someone told you it will help you get your baby 'on a routine'. We'll talk more later about what that actually means and how that might happen. It won't happen by jeopardising your ability to breastfeed.

Are you a bit scared about how breastfeeding might go? I wonder if that's a positive thing. I think it could be. That suggests this is important to you and that's going to help a lot.

The internet can be a good resource too. A website like www.kellymom.com or a website operated by a breastfeeding charity is going to give you access to evidence-based information. You can also read more about the reasons to breastfeed in the first place on the UNICEF baby friendly site. This doesn't mean 'the benefits of breastfeeding' but the 'risks of not breastfeeding'. Find videos that show good positioning such as on Dr Jack Newman's site. If you don't get a chance to see real breastfeeding, it's still all there on video. However some websites are dangerous places so exercise some caution. Is someone trying to sell you something? Is someone speaking from personal experience rather than providing evidence-based information and is that OK? Sometimes it will be. Does what they say fit with the information you are getting from other places?

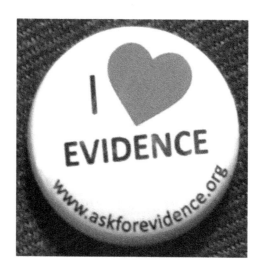

The internet is also the place to find people. Find mums due to give birth at the same time as you and share your journey together. Share breastfeeding videos and resources. Find a parenting board like Mumsnet, Natural Mamas or La Leche League – mother-to-mother forums where people share tips and experiences. Find your tribe on Facebook.

Hopefully your antenatal education will give you some insights into breastfeeding. However an hour is simply not going to cover it. It won't be enough. A couple of hours won't tell you everything you need to know. Expect to need to do some work on your own.

There are four main charities that support breastfeeding families in the UK: the Association of Breastfeeding Mothers, the Breastfeeding Network, La Leche League GB, and the NCT. Why not find out now which charities are particularly active in your area? You can find out who your local breastfeeding counsellor is. They can tell you about local drop-ins. They can talk about which cafes are particularly breastfeeding friendly (though all are required to be by law). It's also a good idea to go along to a support group and chat to some breastfeeding mums and see some breastfeeding. No one is going to think it's weird for a pregnant woman to turn up. They are all going to think you are incredibly sensible.

Get your soldiers lined up. You know where the local breastfeeding counsellor is. You know where the drop-in group is. You know where the local peer supporters are. Ask your midwife who she recommends to support with breastfeeding. How much support can you expect after the birth? Ask challenging questions. What is the reputation of the hospital you are going to give birth in when it comes to breastfeeding? Do they have an infant feeding specialist on staff and a lactation consultant? What hours are they available? Ask these questions now. You want to create an A4 sheet of paper with all the contact details for your team laid out. This is not information you want to start to research if breastfeeding starts not to go to plan. By then you are going to be tired and desperate and have other things to keep you busy.

When you go to hospital, take your feeding plan with you as well as a birthing plan. We'll talk more about what goes on this when we talk about the first hour and first day after birth.

Talk to your support network. Make sure your partner is informed about breastfeeding. They should be watching the videos too. Latching a baby onto a breast is a 360 degree affair and having an extra pair of eyes can be incredibly useful. They need to know why breastfeeding matters and the best ways to support you. Does your partner need to give a bottle and feed the baby in order to bond with their child? Research is very clear that they don't. Once breastfeeding is established there may well be a place for a bottle here and there or even every day, but let's not potentially mess up early breastfeeding success by doing it too soon. We'd only want to introduce a bottle once breastfeeding is well-established and you and your baby have really got the hang of latching and positioning.

The use of artificial nipples is like a master class in bad breastfeeding. You are teaching your baby to associate milk transfer and suckling with an insufficient gape and a retracted tongue position. We want to instil the opposite lesson. More on bottle feeding a breastfed baby later.

If your mother or mother-in-law didn't breastfeed, it can be worth talking to them in pregnancy about your intentions. There are leaflets directed at grandparents and books that they might want to read too. They might not know that it's normal for a breastfed baby to want to feed even though they only fed an hour ago. Or that a breastfed baby might cluster feed in the evenings and feed continually for a block of time even though breastfeeding is going well and mum's supply is great. They might not know that it's normal for a mum's breasts to feel quite soft after the first few weeks and that doesn't mean there is anything wrong. They might not realise that the best way they can help is not by offering to feed the baby but by taking the baby after a feed so you can nap and promising to wake you if they need to feed again.

If someone wants to buy you a gift for the baby, how about a session with a lactation consultant in your home to review your breastfeeding and answer any questions? That may end up being more valuable than even the loveliest stuffed penguin.

The women who are informed about breastfeeding and get the right support usually do make it work if they want to. The scientific fact is that there is a very small minority of women who can't physically breastfeed. Let's talk more about those women.

When many of us were born, our mothers gave birth at a time when breastfeeding rates were the lowest they had *ever been in human history*. Our mothers were often told, 'They didn't make enough milk' because they were being told to feed every 4 hours. My mother-in-law says she wasn't 'allowed' to feed overnight in hospital and the screams of the babies from the nursery weren't exactly conducive to a restful post-birth atmosphere. Mothers weren't given the chance to develop their milk supply and only a tiny minority were lucky enough to succeed in the face of universal sabotage. If we spend the first few weeks feeding in response to our baby's cues, we give our breast tissue a chance to grow and milk supply to develop and all our clever prolactin hormone receptors to form; we give ourselves a chance. It may be difficult for our mums and mums-in-law to see us do things differently and sometimes we need to educate them too.

Who really struggles? A small minority (perhaps around 1%) have what we call breast hypoplasia. This means insufficient breast tissue development. Your breasts may not have changed in puberty and not changed in pregnancy. You may have very widely-spaced breasts perhaps with no noticeable tissue or some tissue but very tubular breasts which bulge into a large areola at the end. If you are not sure whether this applies to you, find a lactation consultant now and ask them. Even if it does, it does not mean you cannot breastfeed at all – just that you need extra help or you may need to supplement your baby with other milk.

Some women may have a hormonal condition such as PCOS or a history of low progesterone. For about a third of women with PCOS, low supply might be a problem. But two thirds of women with PCOS either have oversupply or a normal milk supply! We may not know until we try breastfeeding and find out. Some women with hormonal issues take medications in pregnancy that can aid breast tissue development. If you have a thyroid condition, it's important your thyroid levels are carefully monitored after birth as they can significantly impact on lactation. Have a chat with a lactation consultant or a doctor at the start of your pregnancy.

Some women might think that they have the 'wrong' nipple shape. I've seen babies feed happily on inverted nipples, completely flat ones and nipples longer than a postage stamp (a large letter version). There's a lot of normal. Babies feed by getting a big mouthful of breast and with the right positioning and attachment, it all looks pretty similar. If your nipples are truly inverted, there are some tips that can help. Have a look at the appendix.

Worried your breasts are too large or too small? Large breasts are about fat content rather than glandular tissue and plenty of people with 'A' cup breasts have breastfed happily and successfully. If someone has a smaller amount of glandular tissue, they may have what we call smaller storage capacity. This doesn't mean that their baby will receive less milk overall in a 24-hour period or their milk supply will be low, it just might mean that they need to feed a bit more frequently than their friend with the large storage capacity. However you can't predict these things by looking at the breast from the outside and unless you have some ultrasound equipment to hand, it's better not to try and guess what might happen. If you're worried that your breasts are too large and will be difficult to manoeuvre, breastfeeding counsellors can help with that too.

Taking a medication that you've been told is incompatible with breastfeeding? You'd be amazed how often mothers are told that incorrectly. Drugs manufacturers are often reluctant to pay for the licences and studies than guarantee drugs are safe for a breastfeeding mum so it's easier just to tell mums to speak to their doctor. Doctors can also struggle to find information and are nervous about taking responsibility so it's easier just to tell mums they can't breastfeed. Contact the 'Drugs in Breastmilk' service Facebook page or email druginformation@breastfeedingnetwork. org.uk and check with someone who really knows the research. Have a look at some of the information sheets about medication on the Breastfeeding Network website: http://www.breastfeedingnetwork.org.uk/detailed-information/drugs-in-breastmilk/. Incidentally, there are many mothers who need to take antidepressants and do so alongside breastfeeding with no risks to their babies. Antidepressants and breastmilk is a well-studied area and there is a lot of data available.

Really truly, we've just been talking about a very small group of women for whom breastfeeding doesn't work for physical reasons. We wouldn't be here as a species if breasts failed as often as our culture might lead you to believe they do.

*We wouldn't be here as a species if
breasts failed as often as our culture
might lead you to believe they do.*

Of course, some babies don't always have the necessary tools. Some babies are born with cleft palates, or tongue ties (more on this later). Some babies experience a difficult birth where a lot of medication was used and perhaps they had an assisted delivery that meant the use of forceps and ventouse. That might mean breastfeeding gets off to a tricky start and it's worth being prepared for some of the things that might crop up.

Your Birth

The birth experience is not always something you can entirely control. You can be as ready as possible and as well-informed as possible but sometimes things just need to go with the flow. After you've given birth, the ideal is that baby is placed on your tummy (or higher if the umbilical cord lets them get that far). The baby isn't washed or separated from you unless absolutely necessary. Ideally we let the baby perform a 'breast crawl'. The newborn has an incredible ability to find the breast and latch on all by themselves. They scoot up the mother's body and are guided by smell and primitive vision and find what they need. These instincts might be affected if they have had any intervention or were dealing with medication in their system. Spend some time on YouTube watching breast crawl videos and I defy you not the utter the occasional "Whoah!" http://www.youtube.com/results?search_query=breast%20crawl&sm=3

Send some breast crawl videos to your partner at work and I guarantee the chances of a 'Whoah!' or 'That's coooool!' text are high.

Whether we let baby do their thing, or whether we give them a helping hand, we would aim to have some skin-to-skin as early as possible and plan to try to do the first feed within the first hour after birth.

*Skin-to-skin is also really important
because it means your baby gets
introduced to millions of your very
best friends – the friendly bacteria that
colonise your skin and are
unique to you.*

Skin-to-skin is magic. We know that babies who spend at least that first hour on mum's bare chest are significantly less stressed after the birth experience. Their breathing and heart rate are more stable, they are more settled, and when they are start to breastfeed, they do a better job. We don't really want mum and baby to be separated. Weighing, washing and wrapping baby can all wait. We are learning more and more about the importance of keeping mum and baby together and in skin-to-skin contact at the start of their new life together.

Skin-to-skin is also really important because it means your baby gets introduced to millions of your very best friends – the friendly bacteria that colonise your skin and are unique to you. When a baby comes into contact with YOUR friendly bacteria (which hopefully they did during the birth experience too) their immune system is strengthened and they have a much better chance at fighting off the less friendly infections.

After the first hour, babies seem less alert and may want to sleep for a block of time so we have a useful window to get that first breastfeeding happening. That first feed can happen in a hospital bed, in a birthing pool, in the recovery room after a C-section, on a sofa after a home birth.

What should that first feed look like? There are lots of ways to position a baby at the breast and there isn't one correction position although lying back is a good idea. You certainly don't have to sit up straight to allow the milk to flow and early breastfeeding is best done lying down or reclining. Have a look at www.biological nurturing.com for some ideas.

There are some key principles though. Your baby will need to open their mouth wide: 'the gape'. They need to take a big mouthful of breast and not just to perch on the nipple with pursed lips. The big mouthful of breast gives their tongue a chance to scoop a big chunk of you towards the back of their mouth and get your nipple in the correct position nearer the back of the hard palate.

Feel the roof of your own mouth with your tongue. If breastfeeding is going right, the end of your nipple will sit surprisingly far back along the hard palate and nearly at the soft palate. The end of the nipple will move slightly in space and not rub against anything. If it's going wrong, your nipple may rub against the hard palate or back of the tongue and will get sore. If a nipple comes out looking compressed, squashed, with a white line across it or tapered at the end like an old lipstick, that's a clue something is going wrong.

Your baby needs a big mouthful and ideally more of a mouthful below the nipple than above. We don't really want the nipple to enter the mouth centrally but asymmetrically, nearer the roof of the mouth. Picture that nipple heading where we want it to go, towards the junction of the hard and soft palate. You might think, but if I put the nipple nearer the top half of the mouth how will it go back far enough? Won't it get jammed on the roof of the baby's mouth? Nope. The key thing is giving the tongue as much space on the breast as possible. Then it can scoop as much breast as possible. The nipple will actually be stretched to two-and-a-half to three times its natural length when feeding. It will be extended by that tongue scoop and negative pressure created by the suck.

We need the big gape. But there's no point in having a big gape if other things aren't right too. The baby's chin needs to be making contact with the breast and even more than that, usually pressed into the breast a little. This means that the baby's head will probably be slightly tilted. When you are taking a big bite out of an apple or a burger, you'll usually lead with the chin and lower jaw. Usually the chin makes contact first with the breast. The nose will probably only rest very lightly on the breast or may not even touch at all. Some women with very large soft breasts find that the baby's nose is slightly buried in too. Don't panic. Baby nostrils are very clever. They are designed to leave little air gaps around the corners even when the nose is making complete contact. You do not need to push your fingers into the breast to move the breast away so they can breathe. That's a great way to get blocked milk ducts. Many of our ducts are quite close to the surface of the skin and pushing into the breast with a finger is enough to prevent flow. Try first encouraging your baby's chin to tilt more into the breast. If the baby's nose is still buried, it might just be about the consistency of your breast. The baby will prioritise breathing and come off if there's a problem. That's one reason we don't hold the baby on the back of their head or put pressure on the back of their head. We need to give them the freedom to be able to come off. Holding the back of the baby's head firmly to push them onto the breast can cause a baby to become quite distressed. It may even lead to breast refusal.

The baby's bottom lip will ideally be a bit flanged out. A bit like a fish lip. This gives the tongue more chance of being where it needs to be, over the gum ridge and scooping breast tissue. If the lip is tucked back, the tongue is probably not far out enough. The top lip doesn't need to be flanged out. In fact if the top lip is, that can be an indication the gape isn't wide enough. However here's a thing: once the baby is on the breast and feeding we can't check lips and latch anymore! If a baby is positioned properly we probably can't even SEE the lips and the cheeks are hiding them by making close contact with the breast. If you can see lips or see breast tissue moving in and out of lips, your baby may not have enough breast in their mouth. Be a bit wary if someone wants to check your latch by pulling at your breast or pulling baby's cheeks. Best to check latch by watching as the baby goes onto the breast, watching how they naturally feed, talking to mum about how it feels and looking at the shape of the nipple once it comes out of the baby's mouth.

- *So we've got the big gape.*
- *The more-of-a-mouthful-below-the-nipple.*
- *The chin contact and chin driving into the breast with a head tilt.*

The baby's body should also be in a line. That's to say ear, shoulder and hip all facing the same way. Try drinking a glass of water with your neck twisted to one side.

Baby will also be close and tight to your body if we've got a hope of getting that chin close enough. Rather than just focusing on the 'nose to nipple' which is a message we'll often hear, focus on getting that chin nudged into the breast.

What's happening with their hands? In the early days, hands can seem a little inconvenient. However they are an important part of a baby's sensory tools and help the baby anchor their body so we try and avoid swaddling when breastfeeding and soon the hands will be our friends. Ideally a baby won't be wearing any clothing at all or be wrapped in anything when they have that first feed. You might have a sheet or blanket lightly around both of you. In the early days, if a baby can't get their face to the breast, they'll try and get there with their hands. We don't want the hands to end up on the baby's chest or tucked at their neck as this will push their upper chest away from you which pushes the chin away which means a shallower latch. Baby's hands shouldn't be between your bodies. We also don't want bulky clothing between you or bras containing breast pads squashed between you. One of the reasons skin-to-skin is so great for breastfeeding is you don't have to deal with all the unhelpful fabric in the way! When we recline and babies are on their tummies to feed, it's even more likely their arms will calm as they will feel stable and safe.

What about holding your breast? Hmmm. Be careful about this. A leading cause of nipple soreness and damage is a mum holding her breast and 'offering' it towards the baby or 'putting it in'. Nooooo. The breast is then going to slip subsequently and spring back to its natural position and too much of the nipple probably end up on the hard palate. And holding breasts is a great way to end up with those blocked ducts again. Not to mention the fact that you'll be doing this breastfeeding lark for a lot of hours and you're going to appreciate having a hand free. Be wary of anyone who tries to 'help you out' by holding your breast or touching your baby. None of that should be needed. Some people do benefit from holding their breast but this really won't be everyone and when it happens, it needs to happen minimally and carefully. Sometimes it's better to support a breast that needs it with a ball of socks or a rolled up flannel than by using a hand that can wobble around.

There's a phrase we use a lot: 'baby to breast'. That means that the baby moves TO YOU. You don't move to the baby. Find yourself a comfortable position with good back support and the baby moves to you. If you lean forward, push the breast about, lift the breast up, you are risking problems. If you don't feel you can move the baby towards the breast, check how you are holding them. Perhaps you're holding them just around the head and it feels a bit like your yanking them from the ears? Look at placing more of their body on your arm if you're using the cross-cradle or cradle hold. If you feel the need to lift the breast, are you using a breastfeeding cushion/pillow that's too high? We all have a different amount of space between our lap and our breasts. Breastfeeding cushions perpetuate a myth that we're all roughly the same shape. For some women, a commercial breastfeeding pillow will be far too high. Their breasts hang such that the baby need only rest on their lap. For some people, it's far too low. They also perpetuate the myth we should be breastfeeding by sitting upright. If we lean back slightly, the baby's weight will be resting on our torso and we should not need a cushion at all. Also look at the angle of our nipples. Some of us have nipples that come out at right angles from our body. So baby will come towards our body at a right angle. However a lot of us have nipples that point down slightly, so baby will need to come slightly up from under the breast to make sure both cheeks are making contact with their breast. They will be looking slightly up towards our shoulder, rather than towards the middle of our backs. If we put that baby to the slightly drooping nipple at a right angle, their bottom cheek wouldn't be making contact and some breast tissue on the lower side wouldn't be far back enough in the baby's mouth. Try and breastfeed with your breasts in their natural shape and things will be a lot easier.

So:

- *Big wide gape with bottom lip out like a fish lip.*
- *The more-of-a-mouthful-below-the-nipple.*
- *Chin contact on the breast and chin driving into the breast with a head tilt.*
- *Baby's body close and tight to yours.*
- *The baby's body should be in a line: Ear/ shoulder/ hip.*
- *Baby to breast, not you leaning forward and 'offering'.*
- *Breast in its natural shape wherever possible.*
- *Both cheeks touching breast. Lips not even visible.*
- *Mum comfortable.*

That's too many things to make a clever mnemonic out of. BMCBBNCC?

What will it feel like?

It feels like a teeny being sucking your nipple to about three times its natural length and then massaging your breast with its tongue while creating a vacuum and wiggling its chin up and down.

However that doesn't quite capture the magic.

It feels exciting and important. It feels like this

tiny person is connected to you in ways you couldn't quite imagine. Oxytocin hormone is flying everywhere and you feel quite blissful. Some people say powerful. Perhaps a bit tired too. Exhilarated and peaceful – you can be both of those things at once. The beginning of a really important journey. Perhaps the most valuable journey of your life.

Hopefully a baby doesn't have to come out and start that life before they're ready. Induction is more likely to lead to a cascade of interventions and an assisted delivery so if someone tells you an induction is necessary, do some reading of your own and ask them to provide some evidence. First pregnancies will often naturally extend by ten to fourteen days beyond forty weeks. That isn't necessarily a cause for concern. A baby being delivered by forceps or ventouse may have some bruising that affects the cranial nerves and this can impact on early breastfeeding skills.

There will be times when a C-section is necessary and life-saving. There are also times when a vaginal birth would have been a preference and a possibility. Mothers who do give birth by C-section may need a bit of extra help finding comfortable positions in which to breastfeed. They may not be able to lift baby without help and will need constant care. There is also evidence that mothers who have a C-section may have a delay to their milk 'coming in' (the arrival of their mature milk after the initial few days of colostrum). The reason for this is not always clear but it's particularly important that C-section mums get to do an early feed, ideally within the first hour. This can happen in the recovery room immediately after surgery. Mum and baby need lots of skin-to-skin. And we need to make sure baby is latched on really well and transferring milk effectively so the breasts get the best signals possible. However, despite some extra hurdles, there is NO reason why a mum who has had a C-section won't be able to go on to breastfeed successfully and happily. It may just take a little extra support and determination. By the way, if mum really isn't able to do skin-to-skin for medical reasons then it's time for dad (or partner) to take his shirt off and get on with the job.

When we take pain relief in labour, we sometimes find that baby doesn't arrive quite tapped into all the ideal natural instincts and reflexes. Baby might be drowsy or uninterested in latching on.

Am I saying, "Don't use any pain relief!" Or "Always avoid a C-section!" No, of course not. No one is ever going to be that stupid. Those are your decisions to make with your health care provider. However it's sensible to be informed about how breastfeeding might be affected and what you might need to do to compensate for any early difficulties. If we know that the use of pain relief can delay the 'coming in' of milk or the establishment of breastfeeding in the first 24 hours (which research tells us), then we compensate for that as much as we can with frequent feeding to the baby's cues and checking our baby is attached to the breast really well. Sometimes when your birth doesn't go quite to plan, successful breastfeeding can seem particularly special. If we are anticipating a C-section or a birth with intervention, then we may want to read more about antenatal expression of colostrum so we have some syringes of spare colostrum in case early breastfeeding doesn't go to plan.

We want that good first feed coating the baby's gut with precious colostrum and immediately beginning their protection from disease and allergy. Colostrum is the 'first milk'. We start to produce it at the beginning of the third trimester in pregnancy. Some women notice something that looks like yellow encrusted fluid on their nipples. Some may even notice some leaking. If you don't notice anything, that doesn't necessarily mean early breastfeeding isn't going to go well or something is wrong so don't panic. Some women choose to hand express small amounts of colostrum when they are pregnant as a safety net in case something goes wrong with early breastfeeding. This is called antenatal expression and is often done when there is a higher risk the baby might need to receive formula supplements – perhaps when mum is diabetic and we're concerned baby might have low blood sugar. If mum has some syringes of stored colostrum, we can give that to the baby and keep the baby exclusively breastfeeding. We know that just introducing one bottle of formula can impact on a baby's protection against disease and allergy. We could be sensitising a baby against cow's milk protein. We could be killing off the ideal gut flora environment that gives them better protection against pathogens and allergens entering their blood stream. We could be increasing their risk of a disease called necrotizing enterocolitis. Sometimes, we may need to give a baby some supplementary feeds and that's the best thing for baby. The first rule is 'feed the baby'. However our first choice would always be to do so with mother's freshly expressed milk, then her previously expressed milk, then donor human milk. All those options are ahead of formula.

After that first feed, we may find baby continues to want to feed every few hours or they may have one longer block of sleep and then show interest again. After that first sleep, they then will need to feed roughly 8-12 times in 24 hours. There is a big range of normal when it comes to newborn feeding. Colostrum feeding can be all of the following: twenty minutes every three hours, ten minutes every hour, forty-five minutes every three hours, forty minutes every ninety minutes. And a bunch of other variations. It's very difficult to make rules about breastfeeding when it comes to frequency and length of feeds because babies and breasts are different. We know from one Australian research study that the average number of milk ducts in one group of women was nine. One woman had six and one woman had eighteen. Do we think those mothers will be breastfeeding in exactly the same way?

Be wary of anyone who says to you, "All breastfeeding babies MUST feed for twenty minutes," or, "Must only feed from ONE breast," or, "Must ALWAYS feed from two breasts." Usually we keep a baby on a breast for as long as they are getting value from being there and we'll let them decide. When it comes to colostrum feeding, often we will be offering the second breast but the feeding pattern may change once mature milk comes in and we'll discuss that further later on.

How do we know if a baby wants to feed? You'll hear people talking about 'hunger cues'. A hungry baby that is crying is at the end of a long process of communication and signalling. We're going to try and feed them well before we get to the crying stage as that means we can latch on more calmly. We're learning a new skill and that takes time. A young baby will start to get a bit wriggly when they begin to get hungry. They may move their head from side to side as if they are looking for something. They are. It's you. They may also stick their tongue out and open their mouth a little. They may munch down on anything nearby: their hand, someone's shoulder. They may make little noises.

If you're not sure if they are hungry or not, why not offer the breast anyway? It's much better to get it wrong that way round than miss feeding a hungry baby.

You'll hear people talking about 'feeding on demand' and 'feeding to a baby's cues' or 'responsive feeding'. That is the ideal. Ideally a healthy baby will let you know when they need to feed and when they need to come off. But sometimes we may not always let a baby take the lead. If a baby has had a complicated birth, they might need a bit of a prod. If a baby is jaundiced, we need to make sure they get enough feeds so they can produce enough poo to start getting that bilirubin out of their system. If there are any question marks, we may aim to feed a baby at least every three hours. That means three hours from the beginning of one feed to the next. Let me make that clear, that's not an aim in terms of an ideal. That's the minimum. If a baby wants to feed more than that and showing their hunger cues, that's fine. However if a baby is very sleepy, we'll wake them up and try very hard to get them to feed. If a baby is sleepy, we might take off some clothing and try and cool them down or change their nappy. If a baby latches on but then appears to fall straight to sleep again, we could try using a technique called 'breast compressions' (search on line for a useful video and hand out from Dr Jack Newman). This is a way of getting milk into a baby and encouraging some swallowing and sometimes that will then perk them up and get them breastfeeding on their own. Sometimes the taste of the milk will get them started and trigger their sucking reflex. If they won't even latch on all, there are some things we can do to encourage them. Skin-to-skin is really important for both of you. You could use a little bit of hand expression to get milk flowing and drip some milk into their mouth. A young

Your baby is a teeny-weeny primate. They think they are still connected to you. They want to smell you and be near you and taste you. The prospect of being in a little plastic box, even just a few inches away, is not their first choice.

baby may have one block of four or five hours between feeds but if every block is that long, they may not be getting what they need and you are more likely to get engorged which can cause problems.

Hand expression isn't always obvious. It's not just a case of squeezing a bit. Have a look at some videos online. Look for something called 'Marmet hand expression'. We would ideally prepare the breasts with some warm compresses. Have a go after a shower or bath. Then perhaps do some breast massage to help stimulate milk flow: circular movements around the back of the breast and stroking movements down towards the nipple. Then form your hand into a C shape and cup them around the areola. Thumb one side and fingers the other. Place your fingers about 2cm away from the nipple and feel around the edge of the areola. Compress your fingers together. You may notice some drips forming on your nipple. Try again: opening your fingers again, pressing back into your chest wall, then closing your fingers together and squeezing your breast as it moves forward again. Try and get into a rhythm and the milk should start to flow more easily. If it doesn't, do some experimenting with where you place your fingers or how your squeeze – it's a little different for everyone.

Hopefully you won't need any of that because baby will latch on and feed. How do you know when they are getting enough milk? First of all, what are they doing at the breast? When a baby is feeding from colostrum, you may not hear big glugging swallows but you will still see some evidence of a swallow and chin movement is a good way to tell. When a baby swallows, you will see the chin move down as they create a negative space to draw in some milk and then they bring the chin back up again. They need a little pause before the chin goes back up in order to swallow. The chin movement and tiny pause is a clear indication. The other indication is what is coming out the other end. In the first 24 hours, you will see at least one pee and one poo. The poo will be that sticky tarry meconium stuff. When breastfeeding is going well, it starts to get flushed out. On day two, you'll see at least two poos the size of a £2 coin or bigger. And two pees.

Your First Night

The first night in hospital can seem a bit overwhelming. Where will baby sleep? You may find they want to sleep on someone rather than separated. That is remarkably normal. Your baby is a teeny-weeny primate. They think they are still connected to you. They want to smell you and be near you and taste you. The prospect of being in a little plastic box, even just a few inches away, is not their first choice. We are told that the safest place for baby to sleep is in the same room as you for at least the first six months. That would ideally mean that they are in a Moses basket next to you. Unfortunately not many babies have read the leaflets on this. They'd much rather be snuggled up on dad's chest or in your arms and even attached to your breast. Some families end up bed-sharing, even in that first night in hospital. If that's a possibility, it's important to think through how to do it safely. It's not recommended to bed share if anyone has consumed alcohol (admittedly this may be unlikely just after you've given birth!) nor if either of you smoke. That means even if you smoke outside of the home. A breastfeeding mother sleeping next to her baby tends to take up a protective position. Baby will be sleeping on their back and mum will be on her side with her body curled around the baby and her knees up. A baby doesn't need to wear a hat and we need to check they won't be too warm. You won't be sharing bedding. You may find the hospital has the option of a sidecar crib where the baby can be touched and comforted without mum needing to get out of bed at all. Usually that first night isn't really a 'night' at all. Your baby isn't really born with a sense of day or night. You'll be grabbing naps in an environment that contains unfamiliar sounds and unfamiliar people. The staff may have more on their plate than you were expecting. You (or your partner) may have to go and ask for extra support with breastfeeding.

'Second night syndrome' is also a recognisable phenomenon when baby is experiencing sensory overload. If you are still in hospital, the constant disturbances and stimulus can start to become a little overwhelming. You are tired and baby is also struggling to process their new environment. As Jan Barger, an IBCLC who has studied the second night says, baby wants to go 'home'. You are their 'home' and you might find a baby wants to feed constantly and be in close contact. This is when skin-to-skin is really valuable in helping to reduce stress levels for everyone. Frequent feeding is also really helpful as it gets you practising your positioning and attachment skills and research shows it aids the process of your milk 'coming in'. Even if you are already home, baby can still find the first 48 hours very stimulating. It's important to reduce visitors and unnecessary disturbances to really give everyone a chance to focus on snuggling and nesting.

Your First Week

Nappies are a really useful and reassuring way to measure how your baby is getting on. The baby pooing large meconium poos and getting wet nappies and transitioning to paler stools after a few days is giving us a clear indication that things are going to plan. We don't need to be able to measure millilitres of milk to get that information.

Day One:
At least one poo and one pee. The poo is going to be very sticky and tarry. You might struggle to wipe it off but don't worry, it won't stay like that.

Day Two:
At least two poos and two pees. You may see a little bit of blood in the nappy if you've had a girl. They are reacting to hormones flying around but do check with your midwife if you are worried. Sometimes we might see orangey or red dust in the urine but ideally we won't be getting any of that after day three. Don't forget we're aiming not to go for longer than three hours between feeds (from beginning to beginning) and if your baby wants to feed more frequently than that, that's a good thing.

Day 3:

At least three poos and three pees. Poo should be getting lighter now. More green or brown than black and the consistency less tarry and sticky.

Day 4:

Hopefully you'll have felt a change in your breasts by now which indicates your milk is 'coming in'. You may feel quite uncomfortable and engorged. It can sometimes mean that the breasts get a little bit firmer and baby finds latching on not quite so straight forward. Imagine trying to take a mouthful of a beach ball. It can be helpful to hand express a little to make the breasts softer or use a technique called 'Reverse pressure softening' which means pressing your fingers around the areola for a few minutes to indent the tissue slightly and move the lymph fluid away so the areola and nipple can shape more easily. Sometimes with engorgement, cold compresses can help for comfort and help promote lymph drainage. Your breast is not just filled with milk right now. It's also filled with blood and lymph fluid around the breast tissue and developing tissue. Usually engorgement is a problem for around 24-48hrs. Some people suffer more than others. If your baby is a frequent feeder and feeding effectively, you may notice it less.

As the milk comes in, the feeding style may change a little. Your milk takes a while to transition to mature milk. It's not like a flick of a switch. Mature milk contains more fat. When a breast is full of mature milk, the first few swallows will be relatively low in fat (but high in lactose and water content and lots of other important things). As the baby starts to feed more, the fat molecules work their way from the back of the breast and the fat content in the milk starts to rise. We used to use the terms 'foremilk' and 'hindmilk' but we've found those terms are misleading because it implies the breast makes different kinds of milk. Not true. The fat content may be immediately higher if the breast is emptier and a baby is cluster feeding.

How many minutes does it take the baby to reach the fattier milk? That's a false question. The fat content starts to rise gradually from very early on. The fat content will be higher at four minutes, at six minutes, at ten minutes, at fifteen minutes. However it's going to be different for every mother and baby. We all have that different storage capacity so some mothers may store more of the lower fat content milk. We also have different numbers of milk ducts. Babies also feed differently and have different feeding styles.

We can NEVER say that a baby MUST feed more than twenty minutes on the breast to reach the fattier milk. Some babies will effectively drain a breast in eight, nine, ten minutes and that breast is done for that feed. Other babies will still be going at 25-30 minutes. You're going to need to learn what's normal for YOUR baby.

Normal feeding when the milk has transitioned looks like this: A baby comes to the breast (it might take you a couple of times before you are happy with the latch). They start moving their mouth and sucking and you get the let-down reflex also known as the 'milk ejection reflex'. This is when your areola receives the stimulation from baby and sends a clever signal to the pituitary gland in the brain to release oxytocin hormone. This hormone then arrives in the breast and does more clever things to your milk ducts and the muscles around your milk storage areas. Teeny muscles contract and the milk is pushed down the breast. The milk starts to flow. Without the release of oxytocin, the feed is going to be missing a pretty crucial part of the story. It's not gravity that has the milk trickling out of your breast but the force from these muscles contracting and the baby also creating a vacuum in their mouth which draws the milk in. This is why you can be flat on your baby and still breastfeed just fine. Some people actually feel the milk ejection reflex. It can feel like an electrical tingle. It can sometimes even be quite sore. Some people feel nothing at all. Usually we get at least 2-3 letdowns per breastfeed.

The milk arrives and if the breast is quite full (and the milk therefore higher in water content), you'll probably see some very obvious swallows. You'll probably hear them. You'll see baby's chin moving. Then gradually the fat content starts to rise and things begin to change. It'll go from a suck-swallow-suck-swallow to more like a suck-suck-suck-swallow-suck-suck-suck-swallow. And as the fat content rises further it might be a suck- suck- pause- suck- suck- swallow- pause- suck- suck-swallow. Imagine taking little sips of honey or a thicker liquid towards the end rather than a mouthful of thinner milk. Ideally a baby will come off a breast when they are ready. It may be ten minutes or fifteen or twenty or twenty-five or thirty. You'll realise what's right for your baby. However if you saw that feed change in style as the milk thickened, that's a useful indicator. Most young babies will end a feed fast asleep. That's to be expected. Milk contains sedatives. Oxytocin is one. So is cholecystokinin which incidentally cycles after about twenty minutes. This means the levels start to drop and baby may become more alert again and want a second helping. This is sometimes just the moment when a mum is trying to put a baby down in their Moses basket. "Oh no! She's woken up. She didn't get enough," or, "What is it about this bloomin' Moses basket?" Actually the cholecystokinin levels dropped in baby's blood stream and they had a second wind and they could benefit from a bit more milk. All perfectly natural.

You'll also know things are going well because you'll be seeing the nappies you should be and your nipples should be coming out of the baby's mouth a good shape.

Some people will tell you, "breastfeeding should never hurt." This is a tricky one because 'hurt' is a pretty subjective term. What's normal?

It does seem to be the case that even when breastfeeding is going well and the latch is right, some mothers will experience some sensitivity for the first few days. One piece of research suggested this discomfort should start to get easier after around day five. Sensitivity shouldn't mean you experience pain throughout a feed – just the initial 20-30 seconds as the nipple stretches towards the junction of the baby's hard and soft palate. It also shouldn't mean your nipples have visible cracks and damage and that you are dreading each feed. Sore nipples shouldn't be made worse by feeding more frequently if the latch is correct. If you're sore, you may find it's helpful to express some milk onto your breast after a feed. Breastmilk contains antibacterial properties. Some mothers also find cream such as lanolin useful but cream shouldn't be essential for

It does seem to be the case, that even when breastfeeding is going well and the latch is right, some mothers will experience some sensitivity for the first few days.

everyone. If you are experiencing pain throughout a feed and especially if your nipple is coming out misshapen (flattened at the end, squashed, wedge-shaped, tapered at the end like an old lipstick, with a white line across), you need to get positioning and attachment checked. Don't take one person's word for it if you are in pain. If people seem adamant that your latch is OK and you are still struggling, ask your midwife or breastfeeding specialist to check for a tongue tie. This is a condition that is estimated to affect 10% of babies (statistics vary). It basically means that the tongue movement is restricted because the membrane that attaches it to the floor of the mouth (the frenulum) is too far forward or too short or too tight. The baby might struggle to extend its tongue. Or sometimes they can extend their tongue but not lift it up very far from the floor of their mouth. The tongue needs to be mobile to make breastfeeding work. Babies with tongue-tie may slip off the breast or struggle to attach at all or they may attach but take a long time to feed, make a clicking sound or leave mum in pain. If things can't be improved with specialist help with positioning and attachment, then sometimes the frenulum is cut with a pair of round-ended scissors in a simple operation. It doesn't require an anaesthetic and is best done when a baby is as young as possible so they can then relearn how to use their tongue successfully.

Anything that causes you pain needs to be checked. It's not true that breastfeeding is likely to be painful 'for a while' or several weeks. When it works, it hardly feels like anything. Sometimes not even a gentle tugging sensation. Maybe a flutter. Does it hurt now if you suck on the end of your finger and move your tongue against it? Not really. It might hurt a bit more if you were applying a vacuum and stretching soft flesh a bit but not much. If a mum says, "But my baby has SUCH a strong suck," that's sometimes a clue that the nipple isn't in the right place in the baby's mouth. It's really not that strong a sensation. If breastfeeding was that painful and sore nipples the norm, I'm not sure we'd be here as a species. There was a clever advertising campaign a few years ago by a formula company jokingly emphasising sore nipples as the norm. They are not.

That's not to say that a bit of discomfort in the first few days ALWAYS means something is dramatically wrong. It doesn't. It's just worth getting things checked.

When you get home, it's important to expect the first week to be quite overwhelming. You are likely to be tired and you are likely to be feeling quite emotional. Many women experience the 'baby blues' around day three to four. This can also be when our breasts are engorged and it feels like a tough time. It's important to lower expectations about what you are going to be able to manage. If you wear pyjamas all day, that's fine. Make them cosy ones. If this was Tudor times, you wouldn't even get out of bed for fifteen days. In many cultures, you'd be waited on hand and foot for forty days. In this culture, we celebrate the woman who's in Starbucks talking about inflation and the Bank of England two weeks after giving birth. Your job is to feed baby and look after yourself. Your job is not to cook or clean or entertain guests.

Guests can be really damaging if they come too early and they don't behave properly. You shouldn't have anyone come to visit who you are not comfortable breastfeeding in front of. That's a basic rule. These first few days are absolutely crucial when it comes to getting the hang of breastfeeding and just one day that disrupts that can really set you back. Be brave and ask people to stay away until you feel ready. Skype has been invented for just this purpose. If someone really wants to visit, they can come for half an hour and it's their job to do some household task or cook you a meal.

It's even more important to only surround yourself with people who support you emotionally and practically with your determination to breastfeed. When you are pregnant, you should already have talked to the future grandparents and ideally they will know a little bit already about things like growth spurts and cluster feeding. If you allow grandparents to overrule your parental instincts and decisions, you could be fighting a battle for the next couple of decades. I hope you are lucky enough to have family who only make things easier for you. However, if you are one of the unlucky ones, you may have to say sooner rather than later, "I know you mean well but I may not always make the parenting decisions that you did and I hope you appreciate that sometimes the best support you can give is by allowing us to find our own way."

Babies behave unpredictably and we often spend many hours not quite sure what they want. What does that cry mean? Can they really still be hungry? A useful rule of thumb is, if in doubt, why not breastfeed? It means more practice. It means a better milk supply. It means you get to sit down and cuddle your baby.

You can't overfeed a breastfed baby.

You can overfeed a bottle-feeding baby because the milk flows differently and it's harder for them to control the flow and it's all the same thickness and their 'fullness signal' comes too late. On the breast, if a baby really doesn't want to feed, they will move their tongue and jaw in a slightly different way and move into non-nutritive feeding. Great! It calms them, reducing cortisol stress hormone. It releases the 'love hormone' – oxytocin. It regulates their respiratory rate and heart rate. It keeps them warm so they don't waste calories on temperature conservation. It aids brain development. Even if a baby is just 'using you for comfort' or 'using you like a dummy', that has immense value. Don't fall into the trap of thinking breastfeeding is about the transfer of milk alone. It's also about the transfer of calm and love and comfort. If I'd been floating around in some nice warm amniotic fluid and abruptly arrived in the world, it would be a nice place to be. You taste and smell familiar. As far as baby is concerned, you are still one joined being.

Dummies/ pacifiers aren't a great choice too early on. The breast really is the best place to do the comforting. The real dummy. Using a dummy can mean feeds are skipped and they are connected with a shorter duration of breastfeeding. They teach a small gape and incorrect tongue positioning and these really aren't lessons we want happening now while breastfeeding is getting established.

New babies do sometimes want to feed very frequently. When they are cluster feeding, they may have a period of 4-6 hours when they seem to want to feed constantly. This may happen every night for a little while. They may also have a growth spurt where they have a bananas 24 hours and barely sleep and want to feed every hour. This doesn't mean you have low milk supply. It LOOKS like a baby struggling because mum isn't making enough milk but IT'S NOT. Nature is doing exactly what it needs to do. It's giving the baby the drive to want to feed more frequently so the breasts receive just the signals they need to develop milk supply, form breast tissue and change things like fat levels in the milk.

Some baby care books will tell you this is 'wrong'. They might tell you that your baby should be sleeping independently or only feeding every X number of hours. These won't be books written by people who have studied breast anatomy or normal newborn behaviour.

These first few weeks are a blip in your life. You will have had jam and cheese in your fridge for longer than these weeks will last. You eat when you can, sleep when you can, look after yourself when you can and enjoy this tiny new person who has turned your life upside down.

If that other mother from your NCT class has a baby that sleeps for three hours at a time and feeds for exactly the same amount of time and never seems windy, that doesn't mean that's normal for all babies. There's a lot of normal.

Your First Two Weeks

If breastfeeding is going well, we expect a baby to be back up to their birth weight by around two weeks. After that we aim for about 30g a day for the next few weeks – roughly 200g in a week. We expect babies to lose weight in the first few days and to gradually start to put on weight after around day five. We also would hope a baby wouldn't lose more than 10% of their body weight during the weight loss period.

Sometimes after a certain kind of birth, babies might lose a bit more weight initially. When a mum has an IV drip in labour a lot of that fluid goes into baby and that can mean an artificially elevated birth weight. Babies sometimes even end up looking a bit puffy after the additional fluid. These babies are more like to sail quite close or beyond the 10% loss barrier.

We wouldn't want a baby to lose weight a second time. If that happens, try not to panic. The process has flagged up the fact that you need some additional support with breastfeeding. Someone needs to check your latch, check how often you are feeding, check things like you are not taking baby off the breast before they are finished.

By the end of the first week, baby poo should be nice and pale and ideally mustardy yellow. You should see a minimum of three poos in a day and six heavy wet nappies in 24 hours. Pee shouldn't smell unpleasant or have an obvious colour and if you sometimes get a surprise fountain during a nappy change – great!

Poo may be quite liquidy or it might be thicker like peanut butter and appear to have tiny grains or seeds in it. Sometimes baby poo can be different colours. It might be slightly brown or orangey or even green. Green poo can sometimes provoke panic. Dr Jack Newman suggests new parents are issued with sunglasses so they don't become overly panicked by green poo. If you google 'green poo', you'll get to people talking about a 'foremilk imbalance' and confident claims that your baby isn't getting enough of the fatty milk. Sometimes this *might* be true. If a baby is falling asleep at the breast prematurely or a mum is ending a feed too soon, it could occur. If this IS the case, we'll see it reflected in the weight gain. However if a mum is letting a baby stay on a breast as long as they want to and the baby is actively feeding for as long as it wants to (a normal range on one breast might be something like eight to forty-five minutes), it's unlikely a baby would not be getting enough of the fattier milk.

We used to talk about 'foremilk' and 'hindmilk' and you'll still hear people saying things like, "Is the baby getting enough of the hindmilk?" An emptier breast has a higher fat content. The longer the baby spends feeding at the breast, the higher the percentage of fat in the milk. A fuller breast has a lower fat content milk at the start and it takes a while for the fat molecules to start to work their way down from the back of the breast. As with most things to do with breastfeeding, there's a big range of normal. There are some babies in the world who have never fed for longer than ten minutes in their lives and are putting weight on at a rapid rate. There are some babies who actively feed for 20-30 minutes and really need all that time. So fat content will vary according to how empty the breast is and how many minutes a baby has been feeding on the breast.

It will vary at different times of day too. It seems to be that later in the day, lots of mums 'feel emptier' and babies are not swallowing milk in such an obvious way. Baby may seem to want to feed virtually constantly for a block of several hours. This cluster feeding pattern is common when a baby is feeding from an emptier breast which has a much higher fat content. Cluster feeding takes people by surprise but is fulfilling a really important role.

Your First Month

Once your milk has 'come in' and the colostrum is starting to phase out, it actually takes over a week for the mature milk to fully transition. At the start, your mature milk arriving wasn't much to do with you. It was about hormones. When the placenta was removed, it stopped pumping progesterone hormone into your system (the placenta is a big progesterone factory). Without progesterone, the lactation hormones can start doing their work and lactation revs up. Even women that don't breastfeed at all will notice their milk 'coming in'. There are things that seem to help – your birth experience and your early breastfeeding – but hormones are in charge for the first few days. Then things change, we move to local breast control. This means that your supply is controlled by the amount of milk removed from your breast and how feeding is going. The more milk taken out, the more you will make.

Your breasts are like little streams instead. They can never be completely empty and we know from ultrasound research that even the fullest feed only takes out about 70% of available milk. When baby is taking stuff out of the bottom, stuff is being made at the top. When the milk gets fattier, the stream slows down but it never stops completely. A baby may finish a feed because it's slowed down enough that it's no longer worthwhile to be there and they are ready for the other side now, thank you very much. We might think, 'the first breast is empty' but it isn't really completely empty.

As baby removes milk and stimulates the breast, we are sending signals to maximise our supply and form breast tissue. We are still forming breast tissue for the first few weeks post-partum.

You will hear people talking about 'feeding on demand'. It's not a great phrase as it makes it sound like baby is some sort of tyrannical monster 'demanding' breastfeeding. We could also say 'feeding to baby's cues' or 'responsive feeding'. Your baby is a product of millions of years of evolution and they have built-in the perfect method for maximising your milk supply and doing what needs to be done. We are the ones with the watches and the people telling us that baby 'shouldn't' be feeding frequently (based on science that comes from formula feeding schedules in the late 20th century). We should have every reason to trust our baby.

*We never think: 'breasts are
containers that need to fill up and
I should leave them a bit
so that they do'.*

A common call on the helplines goes like this: "When we first got home from the hospital, for the first couple of weeks, baby would just sleep in the evenings downstairs with us. He would sleep and feed sometimes and we sat and relaxed and had some dinner. Now things are a bit different. Baby seems unsettled for a big chunk of the evening and I don't even seem to have time to eat my dinner. I'm worried he's not satisfied. I'm even worried I might not have enough milk at that time of day". This is a common concern for parents of a 2-3 week year old. This is often when cluster feeding and fussy evenings kick in if they haven't already.

Again, nature isn't daft. Baby has this frantic desire for constant time at the breast and feeding time at an emptier breast because that's a really effective way to get your milk supply developed and your breast tissue maximised. It really might mean that they want to feed constantly for three, four, five hours. It's unsettling. Hopefully by now your latch should be comfortable because lengthy feeding episodes shouldn't mean a mum gets sore provided the positioning and attachment is correct. Some babies may want to cluster feed at other times. I hope for your sake it's not 1-4am. Whenever it happens, it is happening for a purpose. From the outside, it may look like a baby not getting much milk. You may not hear big gulping swallows. The breasts may not feel very full. Important stuff is still happening and we need to let nature take its course. That's not to say it's not tough. If you need a break and you need to go and take a bath and someone else comforts baby and

*And just to really freak you out, we
have a thing called 'growth spurts'.*

tries skin-to-skin and develops their own baby skills, that's not going to hurt anyone. However if we try and feed baby another way because, "Oh my goodness, he's fed non-stop for two hours, I can't be making enough milk," is our perception, we're going to be messing with nature's clever plan. This could end up meaning a mother really doesn't make enough milk before too long. From the outside, it LOOKS like a baby not getting enough milk. The baby is fretful, bobbing around, doesn't appear to be swallowing much and your breasts feel fairly empty and floppy. Whenever you feel yourself doubting your supply, stop and ask yourself about nappies and weight gain. Is your baby putting on weight OK? Did they get those six wet nappies in the last 24 hours and at least three poos the size of a £2 coin or bigger? Did they poo even more than that? Then please try very hard not to doubt your milk supply. Look at the evidence. Evening cluster feeds are often when we are feeling tired too and it's easy to start to worry.

Nature wants our newborns to cluster feed and feed on an emptier breast. It's the best way to develop our breast tissue and it's a great way for baby to tank up on really high fat content milk.

Growth spurts can hit at any time. You might get told that there are often big ones from ten to fifteen days or at six weeks but the reality is that they can hit unpredictably at any time in the first few months. Growth spurts are a period of time (usually around 24-48 hours but sometimes a little longer) when things go a bit bananas. Does your baby usually feed every two hours in the day time and perhaps cluster feed a bit in the evening? During a growth spurt, that cluster feeding might extend for a whole day and night. Your baby might sleep for twenty minutes and then want to feed again. They may want to feed every hour for eight hours. What are they doing? You can probably guess it's all about building up your supply to meet your future needs and they are on a mission. It may be a period of time when you don't get much of a break and baby may also not sleep as much as they usually do. It's a tough couple of days, especially if you are not expecting it. Again, from the outside it LOOKS like a baby complaining about low milk supply. Check the nappies.

But if you've been feeding as normal for a while and your latch is fine and you've not taken any medicine, if it feels like your supply has 'suddenly reduced', it probably hasn't

Check the weight gain. It's far more likely that this is a growth spurt than your supply has magically disappeared.

It's actually pretty tricky for anyone's milk supply to magically disappear. There are a couple of medications someone might take accidentally. Flu and cold medicines sometimes contain an ingredient called pseudoephedrine that can impact on supply, decongestants 'dry you up' in more ways than one. Hormonal contraception can also sometimes have a big impact. Somebody who suddenly stops breastfeeding and draining their breasts may notice a difference in supply. But if you've been feeding as normal for a while and your latch is fine and you've not taken any medicine, if it feels like your supply has 'suddenly reduced', it probably hasn't. It's probably about a normal change in baby's behaviour or maybe your breasts are going through their normal shifts. Breasts don't stay hard and full forever. After a few weeks, we start to feel much softer as breasts get cleverer about milk storage and our breasts are less full of blood and lymph fluid. In the early days, many mothers can easily tell which breast has been just fed from as it's so much softer. We can often tell which breast needs to fed from next. That really can all go and it doesn't mean that your milk supply isn't happily and successfully meeting your baby's needs. In fact, it's slightly odd if breasts stay firm and engorged between feeds indefinitely. It's also normal for leaking to get a little less as the weeks go by and the teeny tiny sphincter muscles around the ducts tighten and your supply is regulated more cleverly.

When we are feeling nervous and we haven't yet got into our mummy stride, it's too easy to start to doubt yourself and specifically your milk supply. Think about nappies and think about weight gain. Would we have survived as a species if our milk supply was so randomly vulnerable? This is what our bodies are designed to do.

The main ways it can go pear-shaped are if someone isn't feeding enough or if the positioning and attachment isn't right. If you are sore to the extent you are starting to dread feeding, something isn't right. No one should be sore at all at any point after the first few days.

It's normal throughout the first month for a baby to feed just as frequently through the night as the do throughout the day. It's amazing how many books out there will claim that babies are supposed to come out of the womb with a delightful ability to sleep from 7pm to 7am naturally and if we don't manage to achieve that then we are deficient and flawed as parents. This isn't biology. It isn't true. The focus on trying to get a baby to sleep longer than nature expects them to is something that can send us loopy in the first few weeks and months so we need to know what is likely and normal.

A good place to start is the ISIS website (https://www.isisonline.org.uk/about/) – run by people who know about infant sleep and have studied it in detail. No, sigh, I'm not trying to indoctrinate you into Islamic State Philosophy. This is the Infant Sleep Information source and if being called 'ISIS' helps sleep-deprived new parents remember its name, that's no bad thing. Take a moment to spend time there and find out what is normal and expected. It is not until around three months that babies may start to develop ONE block of around five hours of sleep at night. Continuing to wake every 2-3 hours before then is NORMAL. Having a three month old that might sleep for five hours and then wake every 2-3 hours is NORMAL. Having a baby that continues to wake through the night (more than once) for the first year of life is NORMAL.

http://www.isisonline.org.uk/how_babies_sleep/normal_sleep_development/

Is it easy? Nope. Do we sometimes wish that babies naturally wanted to sleep for ten hours and then wake slowly and keep their voices down until we've had our first coffee? Oh Yes.

Babies wake frequently because it keeps them safe and they are hungry and they want to say hello and they miss us. If we've signed up to this whole baby thing, a sure-fire way to feeling sad is wishing away the first few months and wishing your baby is controllable but as I mentioned at the very beginning, this new little person is here in your life and they are going to change it in ways we can't always control or imagine. If you have a baby who really wants to party all night long, we just have to check a few things. Could they be reverse-cycling? This is when daytime and night-time is reversed. Your baby might want to sleep for long blocks in the day and then at night they are happily wide awake and want to feed more frequently. A baby that isn't reverse cycling may feed relatively frequently but they will fall back to sleep at the end and sleep until the next feed. No partying.

When a baby is relatively young (under two months), it's probably not a great idea to let them sleep longer than three hours in a block during the day. We really would want them to feed within about three hours from the beginning of the feed to the next one. We want long blocks of sleep to happen at night when it fits with our natural sleep patterns. I know we'd want to feed a baby 'on cue' but if they are reverse cycling and very sleepy in the day, it's a good idea to nudge them along. At night, we want to look at our light levels. The hormone melatonin helps set our natural biorhythms. If a baby is exposed to bright light during the night time (and in the few hours prior to night time), that is going to profoundly impact on their melatonin production. Lots of new parents are flicking overhead lights on to change nappies and see how to latch their baby on. It's going to make an impact. It's sensible to expose your baby to light in the day to try and set their body clock. Then at night time, you need to get a night light which is as dimmable as possible. Blue spectrum light is particularly a problem when it comes to melatonin production. Blue spectrum light is produced by televisions, iPads, and iPhones. It's not great for baby's melatonin but it's also not a great idea for yours either.

feeding in Public

We know that feeding outside the home can seem a bit of an intimidating concept when you're just starting out. There are little hands everywhere and a little mouth that bobs on and off. Milk might spray and there might be some crying (you and/or the baby). This is NOT how breastfeeding will feel forever. When I sit in my local cafes, there are mothers breastfeeding and talking and eating and drinking coffee (yes, you can drink coffee). Their baby may not have the cushions they have at home and the chair might be slightly different but it works and no one appears to be crying. In the first week, this might seem impossible. What is it we are worried about? Are we worried about people seeing our breasts and nipples and

You might read newspaper articles about women being asked to stop breastfeeding in cafes and swimming pools. These make newspaper articles precisely because it's not a common occurrence.

our tummies? Ask your partner to take a picture of you while you are feeding. What does it look like from two metres away? It looks like a woman holding a baby. It's not very exciting. If the idea of latching on is the intimidating bit, you can use scarves, slings and aprons. There are lots of options.

You might read newspaper articles about women being asked to stop breastfeeding in cafes and swimming pools. These make newspaper articles precisely because it's not a common occurrence. Most members of the public either don't notice or don't care. If anyone catches your eye, you'll get a warm, friendly smile. Most public facilities and services now understand they would be breaking the law if they discriminated against a breastfeeding mother and go out of their way to be supportive. In England and Wales, The Equality Act of 2010 protects your rights to breastfeed outside the home. In Scotland, the law goes even further. It is a criminal offence.

Giving a Bottle

At some point, lots of breastfeeding families will wonder about giving a bottle of expressed milk. The baby can stay exclusively breastmilk fed with all the health benefits of exclusive breastfeeding and giving a bottle sometimes suits the circumstances of a family. Some people will tell you that if a baby doesn't receive a bottle within a certain window you've missed your chance and the bottle will then be rejected forever by your baby who perceives it as a minion of Satan. I wonder where that research might come from? Where's the evidence-based for that little nugget? You'll also be told that feeding a baby is something other family members need to do in order to bond with baby. As if cuddling, skin-to-skin, bathing, playing are all inferior to the joy of popping a bit of plastic in a mouth. There's no evidence to support that either. You give a bottle when it feels right for you and your family, not because someone has frightened you into it. And you know what? Lots of people never actually feel the need. They breastfeed and mum and baby go out and about and sometimes baby gets left with babysitter and that's all possible without a bottle. And then at around six months, a cup might be introduced. Cups are better for the palate and better for teeth and recommendation is to stop using bottles by around twelve months anyway.

If you do want to give a bottle, it's worth checking that breastfeeding is established. Some people will tell you it's always best to wait for about six weeks but that may not always be necessary. There are three things we need to protect: your baby's latching skills and your supply and breasts (OK, that's four things). A baby feeding from a bottle is having a master class in poor breastfeeding technique. Their tongue is in the wrong position. They are using their tongue and jaw muscles differently. Milk is pouring out with no effort and that's not how things work on the breast. It's worth looking on YouTube for a technique called 'paced bottle-feeding' which helps to slow things down.

If we're using a bottle, let's try and make it as similar to breastfeeding as we possibly can. That doesn't necessarily mean using the bottle claiming to be most like the breast. Most manufacturers will make that claim. Some of them have bottles with extraordinary shapes and elongated nipples. Surely it would be logical to use a bottle that allows the baby to place their bottom lip 'on the areola' just as they do on the breast? We want the baby to have a big wide gape, with their tongue extended over their gum ridge. It doesn't seem sensible to have their lips pursed around the end of a nipple. It's also a good idea to slow things down and keep the bottle as horizontal as possible so that they still need to use some effort and create a negative space to draw milk out. We want to keep a newborn sized hole in the teat and require them to work at it.

When it comes to the amount in the bottle, we need to be careful. The sucking reflex is a powerful thing in a newborn. They will OFTEN overfeed from the bottle once they've got into the flow. We know that bottle-feeding and obesity are connected. It's not completely clear why, as there are various factors, but one theory is that babies feed quickly from a bottle and it comes out so quickly that their 'fullness switch' doesn't have time to go off.

So what we don't do is feed a baby from the bottle and think that reflects at all on what is happening on the breast. A baby will feed normally from the breast and often still want milk from a bottle. That doesn't mean they weren't getting enough from the breast. Bottle feeding is so easy that the act of refusal is likely to take more effort for a younger baby. Young babies want to suck on things! A baby will also often keep going so it's going to be up to us to limit the amount. A month old baby takes on average between 600-800ml of breastmilk in 24 hours. If they feed around ten times in 24 hours, that's going to mean roughly 70ml in the bottle will be needed. The first few times it might be sensible to put less in the bottle so if things don't go to plan, you haven't wasted all the milk. Once you've started feeding, a bottle can be saved for an hour and then would need to be discarded.

We also need to think about what's happening to your breasts in the meantime. In the early days, our supply is still quite vulnerable. When breasts become engorged, we're sending signals to reduce milk supply. We're accumulating a particular whey protein called FIL (feedback inhibitor of lactation) and changing the shape of our prolactin receptors and that tells our body to make less milk. We also know that when new mums skip a breastfeed they are also much more likely to risk getting blocked ducts and possibly even mastitis. It's particularly a bad idea to skip breastfeeds at night time. Between midnight and 5am, our prolactin hormone levels are higher. This is the hormone that governs our milk supply and emptying our breasts at this time is particularly key to developing our supply. If someone is going to give a bottle, ideally you'll be expressing around the same time or just before. You'll want to keep your breasts regularly emptied. That's what helps protect and maintain our supply. When breasts get engorged, not only do we risk reducing our supply, we also increase our risk of mastitis and blocked ducts.

As the name suggests, blocked ducts are sometimes about a physical blockage in the duct which prevents milk flowing freely. Sometimes too much milk gets left behind and leaks out into tissue where it's not supposed to be. The body interprets this as an attack from a foreign body and sends the lymph and white blood cells and we get an inflammation. This can mean a firm tender area in the breast and we need to use warm compresses, massage and frequent drainage to get it cleared. If we can't manage to get the breast back to normal, sometimes bacteria might arrive and the breast can start to look red. We may get a temperature and start to develop flu-like symptoms and that's mastitis. We would continue to use warm compresses, massage and frequent drainage using a variety of positions and methods. If things don't improve within 24 hours, we may need to contact our doctor and get a course of antibiotics. Hopefully none of that is going to happen and you can continue to keep your breasts drained and introduce bottle-feeding happily.

We're going to need something to go in the bottle.

How do we start pumping?

Everyone responds differently to pumping and expressing so it's very difficult to make hard and fast rules. There some key things that are worth remembering. The

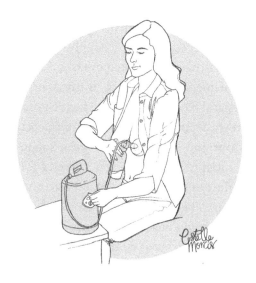

way a pump takes milk out is completely different from the way a baby does. We are trying to fool our bodies into thinking this plastic and silicon and mechanical object is our baby. We trick it into releasing oxytocin, 'the love hormone'. If we manage to get that hormone released then you'll achieve the letdown reflex (or 'milk ejection reflex') and milk will start to flow. PLENTY of people with a generous and healthy milk supply have intelligent breasts not so easily fooled. They may end up pumping very little and incorrectly assume the issue is with their milk supply. Even if we do manage to achieve a letdown reflex, you may only get one in a session when a baby breastfeeding may trigger two or three or even more.

We never use pumping as a way of judging milk supply. You cannot test to see 'how much the baby is getting'. A popular babycare books talks of doing a 'yield test' – to pump to judge how much milk your baby might receive in a particular feed. Stuff and nonsense. There are plenty of women with oversupply who just don't respond to the pump and hardly manage to pump anything while their baby glugs away. Plus the minute you start imagining a pumping session is about measuring your milk supply, it's

We never use pumping as a way of judging milk supply. You cannot test to see 'how much the baby is getting'.

very likely you'll be getting stressed and inhibiting your oxytocin release – the hormone we need to get the milk flowing and the 'letdown' reflex happening.

If you do struggle to get the letdown reflex happening, it can be a good idea to take a moment to prepare the breasts. The Marmet hand expression technique encourages you to massage the breasts before you start. Have a look online for some videos to see the technique. It can also be a good idea to use some warm compresses before you start or try and express after a bath or shower. You may find that starting with some hand expression before you use the pump or even just sticking with hand expression gets the best results for you.

What type of pump is best? That question can't be answered. Some people get better results with a manual pump that retails for £30. Some people will get more milk out with a double-phase hospital grade electric breast pump that rents for £40 a month and retails for more like £1000.

If you need to do a lot of pumping, it might be sensible getting hold of a hospital grade double electric pump. Being able to pump from both sides at once saves time and helps you to get the milk ejection reflex more easily. You can rent a hospital grade pump from a company like Ardo. If you are going to return to work after only a few months, you may want to spend a bit more on getting a robust double pump so you can save time and also give as much breast milk for as long as possible. If you are only going to pump occasionally or just a few times a week, a personal use consumer grade single-sided pump might suit your needs just fine. Be wary about borrowing old pumps or buying second hand. Some pumps have 'open' systems which means milk can get into the mechanism and they are not intended to be used by more than one person.

Wash your hands thoroughly before you start. You don't need to wash your breasts. Pumping shouldn't hurt. Check that you don't have the suction up too high. Also check that the diameter of the funnel (known as the 'flange) is the right size. Nipples are different diameters and not all pumps are going to work for everyone. If the edge of your nipple is rubbing against the side of the flange when you are pumping (or too much of the breast is being sucked in), you may need to get a differently sized flange and most of the major pump manufacturers can provide that.

Storing milk is something else you're going to need to know about. Breastmilk contains macrophages that eat bacteria. Research shows that a bottle of breastmilk left in a fridge will contain fewer bacteria in it after a few days than it did at the beginning. However breastmilk isn't designed to sit around forever. It's fine at room temperature for about six hours. It's fine in the fridge for up to eight days (assuming your fridge is 4C or below and you don't put the bottle in the door). It's fine in a freezer (below -17c) for six months and a chest freezer for up to twelve months. There's good information about milk storage here: http://www.breastfeedingnetwork.org.uk/ breastfeeding-help/expressing-storing/

Human milk in a bottle isn't homogenised like the cow's milk in your fridge. It will separate and you'll get a little layer of cream on the top while the rest looks a lot like water. When you are in new-mum-paranoia mode, it's easy to worry your creamy layer isn't as thick as it's supposed to be. Human milk doesn't have a particularly high fat content compared to other mammals. Our milk is about 4% fat. Compare that to reindeers at 20%, porpoises at 45% and grey seals at 53%. Other mammals have milk that allows them to feed their baby and then wander off and find a few berries or do a few hours of fishing. We are 'carry mammals'. Our infants are designed to feed frequently. Our milk has the perfect blend of fat, protein and carbohydrates to fuel our complex brains. Unlike a mammal like a cow, we don't have a huge muscle mass. Our milk is right for us.

If your milk has separated, just swirl or shake it back together when it's time to feed. Unless you have a bionic arm, shaking the milk isn't going to do it any harm. It may also be a good idea to warm the milk slightly under a hot tap or by sitting in a basin of hot water. It's not recommended to use the microwave as that can leave unpredictable hot spots. Cold milk means a baby has to use up energy and calories bringing it back up to their body temperature.

Once milk has been defrosted, it needs to be used within 24 hours. Once a baby has started to drink from it, it would need to be discarded after an hour as it's contaminated with saliva.

If you are pumping more than once a day, you really

don't need to continually wash and sterilize the breast pump. Remember that a bottle of breastmilk can sit there on your coffee table for six hours so why are we washing a pump that's only come into contact with milk and pretty clean skin? You can use a technique called 'wet-bagging' where you put the pump in a plastic bag and pop it in the fridge. The next time you use it perhaps use a paper kitchen towel to wipe off the cold drips, otherwise just use it. Washing it once in 24 hours is plenty.

Babywearing

Definition: *Babywearing [verb]: carrying a baby in a soft pouch, sling or wrap – sometimes for several hours in a day. Babywearing is often about a physical convenience but advocates also believe it has an important emotional and psychological benefit to the mother/ baby dyad.*

Why do you think babywearing often seems such a natural step for a breastfeeding mother? Why is it that when you go online the parenting sites that are openly supporting breastfeeding past twelve months inevitably have a membership also passionate about slings and babywearing? It doesn't seem much of a stretch to suggest that when a mother achieves the biological norm of breastfeeding successfully, babywearing naturally follows and is often a part of that instinctive natural parenting.

Babywearing is not fashion any more than breastfeeding is fashionable. As Meredith Small says in her book, "Our Babies, Ourselves": 'during 99% of human history the pattern of infant eating, sleeping and contact was that human infants were carried all the time, probably slept with their mothers and fed frequently throughout the day'.

To promote babywearing and discuss it as the biological norm obviously can make other mothers who choose not to do it uncomfortable or even feel guilty (but we could say the same about many parenting decisions.) There are able-bodied mums who would be perfectly capable of baby-wearing but will instead strenuously support their desire to travel around town with £400 worth of baby tank in the belief this is more 'convenient'.

A Bugaboo Cameleon currently retails at Mothercare for around £850. For that price, you could get a decent sling and actually hire someone else to walk alongside you carrying your baby for you.

When a baby wants to be constantly held our society tells us something is wrong. Mothers can create 'rods for their own back' with constant attention. Even in the 21st century, people talk of how you can spoil a baby by holding it too much. When we trust baby and trust our own maternal instincts to hold, to respond to cues – breastfeeding is more likely to succeed and humans fit their evolutionary expectations.

For support with babywearing and to try out some different slings, visit your local sling library or sling meet: http://www.slingmeet.co.uk/. You can also get lots of information about types of slings and where to buy them at www.thebabywearer.com.

And slings can be really pretty too!

Your Second Month: Routines

Once breastfeeding is up and running (it doesn't hurt, baby is putting on weight, you are all surviving), a lot of people find themselves looking around and thinking, "Right, what's next? What should we be doing now?"

In our culture (this pocket of Western industrialised post-WW2 civilization), the big message is 'your baby should be on a routine'. They are supposed to be predictable now. You are supposed to know when they are going to feed and sleep. It's your job to get control.

We often get these messages from our older relatives who were parenting when babies were put in prams for naps at set times and if they didn't sleep, hard luck. Or were parenting at a time when breastfeeding rates were at an all-time historic low and bottle feeding patterns were rigid.

But these messages come from our peers too. Many women now give birth in their thirties after a successful and empowering career. It's very appealing to keep control over life with baby too and be in charge of day-to-day routine. We may not have the family support we once had and we desperately hope that by controlling routines, we can cope with the unpredictability of this tiny new person we spend our days with.

The best-selling baby books are powerfully giving the message that 'routine is king'. Not only is it possible to control when a baby eats and sleeps but it is desirable. If you can achieve it, you are a successful mummy who has tried just that little bit harder. Those mummies still feeding in response to baby's cues at two or three months? Or not always able to pinpoint the start of their baby's nap to the precise ten minute window? Just not following the right 'plan'. Reading the wrong books. Haven't found the holy grail (i.e. their book, not that other book).

New mums are insecure. They are trying to find their way in the world and learning to trust their instincts. They are trying to work out how to be lovers and mothers at the same time. They are trying to make new friendships and discover a new side of themselves. They are incredibly vulnerable when it comes to messages about success and competition and what we're 'supposed to be doing'. It takes a very brave woman to say, "OK, so three of my NCT group are all reading that particular book and claiming it's all about trying to set up a routine but what we're doing works for us. We don't all have to mother in all the same way. This isn't a race."

That particular book will claim that all babies can feed after a three hour interval (or whatever their magic number is). Unfortunately that view shows a basic ignorance of how human biology works and in particular something known as 'breast storage capacity'.

Our knowledge about breasts has been transformed over the last twenty years. Much of the pioneering work has been done in Australia by scientists like Professor Peter Hartmann and Dr. Donna Geddes, Steven Daly and their teams.

We used to think most women had a pretty similar number of milk ducts but the ultrasound research revealed there were less than previously thought and the range was big. One woman had six ducts at the nipple. One had eighteen. (http://www.ncbi.nlm.nih.gov/pmc/articles/PMC1571528/)

But it's the findings about breast storage capacity that we need to talk about here. When a baby feeds, some milk is manufactured during the feed itself and some is taken from milk that has been stored in the breasts between feeds.

Ultrasound revealed that a mother's storage capacity cannot be guessed from breast size. Breast size is obviously not just about glandular tissue. The range in breast storage capacity was huge. One woman stored 80ml and another stored 600ml. (http://mammary.nih.gov/reviews/lactation/Hartmann001/)

Women with a smaller breast storage capacity had a healthy milk production over a 24 hour period and their babies had good weight gain. But their babies might need to feed more frequently to access this healthy milk production. Over the entire 24 hours, the baby with a mum with larger storage capacity received 956ml. A baby whose mum had smaller storage capacity received 896ml.

Is this a mother with a supply problem? Clearly no,

it is not. Her baby may continue to feed two hourly or even less for a few months during the day, cluster feed at certain points and perhaps continue to wake a couple of times hungry at night. Her friend's baby may settle into a pattern of feeding less frequently over a 24 hour period. Both have good supply and normal breastfeeding experiences.

When breasts are fuller, milk production slows. When breasts are emptier, we make more milk. When babies feed more frequently and from emptier breasts, they receive milk with a higher fat content. Frequent feeding has value. And as human milk has a fat content of around 3-5% compared to some mammals who have a fat content of 40% +, it seems pretty clear we're designed as a species to need feeding more frequently.

But let's imagine the mother with the smaller breast storage capacity has read this baby care book. She might become distressed that her baby still wants to feed two hourly. She might even try and stretch the interval between feeds in the mistaken belief this will increase her baby's intake. And in doing so, her breasts spend longer at full storage capacity and their milk production slows and her breasts receive the signal to decrease milk supply.

So in her attempt to stretch between feeds as the advice she is reading suggests she does, she may actually be decreasing her overall milk production in 24 hours and be doing some actual harm.

There are still people out there, surrounded by breastfeeding, who believe that a baby who feeds after four hours rather than three hours will 'take more milk'. There are people who believe that you need to wait and hold a baby off to let your breasts 'refill'. There are people who believe that when a baby does want to return to the breast after only an hour that must reflect a 'problem' and perhaps the mother even has a supply issue.

It's scary and extremely frustrating that basic messages about how milk production works don't reach the people who need them.

You will need to find a breastfeeding pattern that works best for you. Am I saying that if your two month old baby is still feeding every ninety minutes all around the clock, you just have to lump it and wear your 'Earth Mother' t-shirt? No. There are lots of things you can do. You can work on the quality of your latch. You can look at whether you are offering the second breast (or returning to the first one). You can look at using breast compressions or encouraging cluster feeding when it works for you. There are things you can do.

But if your baby doesn't fit what that book says it should fit, that's expected. Babies need to eat and drink at different times for a whole host of reasons just like we do. And I bet the writer who claims babies should only eat every three hours doesn't sit in her kitchen waiting for the clock hands to move so she's permitted to have her next cup of tea.

Just check that if you are busting a gut to follow a baby manual, it's making you happy. These few months will never come again. Your baby is only teeny once and before you know it they are eating mud and kicking balls and eating balls and drawing dinosaurs and learning all the names of Thomas the Tank engine's associates and wearing clippy-cloppy shoes. I know mums who have made themselves sad by trying to make the first year of their baby's life fit a schedule that came from somebody else with no evidence-base to support it and no logical arguments in its favour.

Follow your heart. Don't do what you feel you are 'supposed to be doing' because someone else said that responsive parenting was wrong.

And if you really want to start introducing a routine, don't follow a book like it's a religious tome. Look at what your baby is naturally already doing. Talk to people in your community who are trained and updated about things like baby sleep and infant feeding. Talk about your own personal circumstances. Phone a helpline. Find a method of introducing a routine that is individual to you and your baby.

Research published just recently from Swansea university and Newcastle university confirmed what we instinctively know – that a responsive approach to early

This phase in your baby's life will last for less time than most of us have jars of strawberry jam in the fridge.

parenting protects your chances of breastfeeding. Those introducing strict routines either were less inclined to breastfeed at all or stopped in the first few weeks. If you are under pressure to introduce routines early on, take some time to reflect on your decision before you end up going down a road that may be difficult to return from.

This phase in your baby's life will last for less time than most of us have jars of strawberry jam in the fridge.

Why Stay Exclusively Breastfeeding?

You probably already know that the recommendation of the Department of Health in the UK and the Departments of Health in pretty much every other country in the world is to 'exclusively' breastfeed for the first six months. Then introduce solids alongside breastfeeding and continue to breastfeed for as long as both mother and baby wish.

Exclusive breastfeeding means a baby under six months only receives breastmilk (and medicine if needed). No water is required for a breastfeeding baby even on the hottest day in the summer. And once we give one bottle of formula that baby is no longer 'exclusively breastfed'.

Giving formula is a very personal decision to every family. For some families, with a history of diabetes or family allergies, not giving even one bottle of formula is a priority. We know that it can change the body's response to dairy proteins and can have a long term health impact. For families with a less obvious health issue, it might seem less crucial. If you have the choice not to give formula though, it's worth knowing why 'exclusive breastfeeding' is the recommendation. If you choose to give formula alongside breastfeeding of course your baby still gets tons and tons of health benefits from the breastmilk they receive. Some things are changed though and it's worth knowing a bit more about that. Breastmilk contains a special sugar called an oligosaccharide. It lives symbiotically in the human gut with friendly bacteria and a protective coating is formed over the gut wall. This coating stops pathogens that cause disease and allergen molecules from entering the baby's blood stream. This is one of the reasons that exclusively breastfed babies very very rarely get gastroenteritis and diarrhoea-type infections. This means pathogens pass through the gut without entering the baby's blood stream. Statistics show that babies hospitalised in the first year of life for gastroenteritis and respiratory infection are far more likely to be formula feeding babies.

Many women don't have a choice about whether to introduce formula. It was a decision that was right for them and their family in that moment. The first priority is to 'feed the baby'. Perhaps breastfeeding didn't work out through lack of support. Perhaps they have physical or medical issues. It's not up to us to second guess everyone's decisions. We can only hope that everyone who wants to breastfeed gets to breastfeed for as long as they want to. We can only hope that people don't give up through lack of information or because they couldn't find the right people to help them.

However the decision to perhaps introduce 'the odd bottle of formula' when your milk supply is otherwise fine and your baby is well is something I'd like you to be informed about. If you give formula, you change the Ph.

of your baby's gut and those friendly bacteria that were doing their job of coating the baby's gut wall won't be able to survive. Your baby's gut flora will change and instead of being colonised with things like 'bifidus factor', new bacteria move in. Adult gut bacteria like Colostridium difficile and higher levels of E.Coli and streptococci. This is one reason the stools of formula feeding babies smell different and more similar to adult stools.

Giving a bottle of formula does then reduce some of the protection breastfeeding can offer against disease and allergy. UNICEF estimate that with a modest increase in exclusive breastfeeding rates in the UK, 3,285 gastrointestinal infection-related hospital admissions and 10,637 GP consultations would be averted each year. (http://www.unicef.org.uk/Documents/Baby_Friendly/Research/Preventing_disease_saving_resources.pdf)

You may still feel it's right for you and your baby to use formula and that is entirely up to you. You are going to be making that decision for a bunch of reasons that are about more than gut bacteria. However once your baby's gut 'closes' by around six months, introducing formula is likely to be less harmful as the permeability of the gut is less of a factor and the loss of the friendly bacteria coating less relevant. Plus the introduction of solid food at around six months will change gut Ph. anyway.

I just want you to take a moment before you end exclusive breastfeeding and check you've read some things (not just this) and you feel you are making a decision that is right for you. We live in a society where formula marketing spend a very large sum of money in targeting you. There are people who sit in offices who devote their working day to encouraging you to *not* exclusively breastfeed. Companies want you to feel formula is well-made and contains lots of lovely ingredients and they work very hard in presenting themselves as warm and fluffy – using techniques that take them right up to the edge of UK law and beyond. They want you to sign up to clubs and enjoy your free cuddly toys with their logo on them. They may have talked to your midwives and paid for their training. They really don't want you to take a moment to read about hospitalisation rates and gut flora. They use very clever messages about how formula will help you and how breastfeeding requires sacrifice and the 'perfect' diet. We might all think we are able to resist advertising messages. The infant feeding survey looked at who is using 'follow-on' formula (the only formula allowed to be openly advertised on TV in the UK) and the figures on who is using follow-on under six months (an age group it's not designed for) suggested otherwise. 16% of UK mothers have given their babies follow-on formula at four months old.

You can read more about how the formula companies break the law in the UK to try and get YOU not to breastfeed here: www.babymilkaction.org/monitoringuk17

Your Third Month: Breasts Change

One thing that we can also add to the new-mummy-paranoia-hit-list is how our breasts change once breastfeeding has become established. The early engorgement that we experience in the first few days as our milk comes in isn't expected to last. That engorgement is about our breasts being filled with lymph fluid and blood as well as milk. The body is working hard to develop breast tissue and make changes to your milk. You may also be dealing with fluid left over from your birth if you had a drip.

However even after that first week, our breasts often feel quite full. The body makes milk constantly as it gets used to what baby needs and it constantly gets reabsorbed and re-made. It's usually very clear when a feed is due from how our breasts feel. We may feel quite uncomfortable and we get a sense of relief once a feed has finished. If you are feeding from only one side, it's very clear which breast is due its turn.

After a few weeks, this starts to change. Our breasts get a bit cleverer at making the level of milk made by our baby. We may need less lymph and blood surrounding developing breast tissue. It's actually quite normal to not really be able to tell which breast you are going to feed from next. You may even experience a relatively long interval between feeds without getting too uncomfortable.

At the beginning, people also find leaking quite reassuring and imagine it's an indication of having a lot of milk. We can get nervous when we leak less but this is also very normal as the little teeny sphincter muscles around the duct endings tighten.

You might also be someone who feels the 'milk ejection reflex'. Some people feel this as a tingle or a quite sharp sensation that feels like a jolt of electricity. If that starts to fade, mums can imagine something is wrong and the letdown isn't working properly. Not so.

All these changes are normal. In fact we're more likely to be worried about the mum who IS still feeling very engorged and uncomfortable after a couple of months have gone by. If you are worried that you might have low milk supply, have a look at the section on 'complications'.

Your fourth Month: Sleep

If you go onto google and type in 'four month', note how one of the top searches coming up is 'four month sleep regression'.

I'm really sorry to break it to you but this can be a thing. Sometimes babies are just getting the hang of that nice 4-5 hour block of sleep at night and we are just starting to get used to sleeping long enough that our eyes don't physically hurt in the morning, and then it all seems to go a bit pear-shaped again. We might use the term 'regression' but actually it's a progression. It's a developmental step as babies develop neurologically and physically.

I'm mentioning it in a book about breastfeeding because it's a common misconception that this has something to do with baby not 'getting enough'. You'll even get people to tell you to ignore current Department of Health recommendations and start solids early, well before the recommended six months.

Four month sleep 'regression' is about a number of different factors and it's rarely a reason to end exclusive breastfeeding. Sometimes we do get babies at this age reverse-cycling. That means mixing up day and night. If you are four months old, the world has become a very interesting place. Everything is exciting and stimulating and while breastfeeding is all very nice, it takes you away from THE STUFF. So you'll breastfeed when you are really hungry and thirsty and really need it but often only for the minimum and then it's STUFF TIME. Meanwhile, at night, the stuff is all dark anyway and you can't see it as easily, so you may as well do some nice long feeds then. This is reverse-cycling. Sometimes we can get round this by creating an excitement-free zone in the day. Some people actually black out a room for day time feeds. Some people go completely the other way and make breastfeeding extra fun. You can buy things called nursing necklaces that mum wears around her neck and is filled with chunky interesting colourful things. The idea is that baby will still want to stay breastfeeding as their line of sight at the breast allows them a look at everything on the necklace just perfectly. You also hear of mums breastfeeding four month olds while bouncing on birth balls, singing nursery rhymes and turned to give a view out of the window. All in the name of trying to get baby to take just a little bit more milk in daylight hours.

Four month old babies are also hitting some other developmental milestones. They are much more conscious of their gross motor movement. In the middle of the night, as they transition between sleep cycles, they are more aware of what their legs and arms are doing and fully rouse instead of sleepily transitioning to the next

*One popular babycare book uses the
delightful phrase 'accidental parenting'
– as if following maternal instincts
and showing love and attention
are horrible misfortunes.*

sleep cycle. While they are awake, they might as well check in and ask for a bit of milk. Is that a baby waking for hunger? Not really. But now they've fully roused, breastfeeding is looking pretty appealing.

If you are in the thick of the four month sleep regression, it can be tough because it's normally a time when you are really starting to get out and about – meeting other mums, trying out new activities. Now that feeding is pretty much cracked and you've just worked out how to properly pack a change bag, this seems like a cruel blow. You may need to return to scheduling a little bit of sleep time for you in the day and asking for some help with extra lie-ins.

You'll hear some people worrying that by responding to their baby at night they are creating 'habits'. One popular babycare book uses the delightful phrase 'accidental parenting' – as if following maternal instincts and showing love and attention are horrible misfortunes. The reality is that your baby is going to change again.

This will not be your life forever. One day you will open your eyes in the morning and realise you've been able to sleep all night. It will happen. At six months and at eight months they will be a different little person with different influences and stimulations. Things will change again.

Starting Solids

The Department of Health and the Department of Health of every other industrialised country in the world recommends the introduction of solid food at around six months. You may hear 'rumours' that this will change. You may hear people tell you that there's something wrong with this recommendation and earlier is best. Not true. The recommendation to wait until six months was the result of some careful deliberation and an examination of a wide range of evidence that looked at issues like disease and allergy prevention. There are a few bits of infant physiology that are hard to argue with. Babies need the amylase enzyme to digest starch and it isn't properly released until around six months. In the days when people would spoon rice cereal into their small babies like filling cracks in the wall with polyfilla, some of those nutrients weren't going anywhere useful. Babies are born with what we call an 'open gut'. This means the gut wall which separates the baby's intestines from the blood stream is extremely permeable. Larger molecules that might cause disease and allergic reaction can pass through easily. Breastmilk does a clever thing as it forms a protective mesh over the gut wall that prevents various nasties passing into the baby's bloodstream. However to get that mesh functional we need the baby's gut flora to be the good stuff. Just as if we were going to end exclusive breastfeeding, adding in solids will change the gut Ph. and gut flora and some of that protection could be lost. However by around six months, gut closure has occurred in babies and introducing other food then appears to have less of an effect.

A baby who is six months can also participate much more in the feeding process. They can sit up and hold and bite and select and get that food is colourful and textured and wonderful. They can control the process. Rather than simply be vehicles for beige mush. You'll often hear people say, "But my four month old looks so longingly at us when we eat our bacon sandwiches. He looks so fascinated and he wants to reach out and grab my food. I don't want to make him wait until six months". Sure but the same baby is probably going to look equally fascinated when you apply mascara and lipstick. Probably not the best argument for starting solids ahead of the recommendations.

"My baby is big. He'll need solids sooner." Nope. It's really not the way it works. Our bodies are designed to make enough milk for twins. It can cope with your bigger-than-average baby.

"My baby is smaller. She'll need solids sooner." Nope. If you're concerned about weight gain, there are more effective things we can do to increase calorie content.

"My baby doesn't sleep well. He needs solids sooner." This may well be the classic sleep regression that we discussed at four months. This is not connected to insufficient nutrition. We may even find that introducing solids causes more restless nights initially, not improved ones. Babies are experiencing new digestive sensations, pooing at different times and are more likely to be constipated.

This is one area where we may get a lot of pressure from friends and family. Many of them weaned at a time when the recommendations were different. If you've been breastfeeding, they are probably super keen to get the spoons out and literally get stuck in. You may hear this from your mother-in-law: "Well, Bob had baby cereal from six weeks and he's just fine." Bob now plays rugby, runs marathons, splits atoms – delete as appropriate. The anecdotal evidence argument is never a worthwhile one. Bob is probably a member of a generation with shocking levels of obesity, heart disease and diabetes. Perhaps if Bob hadn't have been weaned at six weeks, he'd play better rugby and split more atoms.

The recommendations didn't change because someone in government had a long lunch and was feeling cross with Heinz baby foods that day. Evidence looking at the health of babies breastfed for three to four months vs six months was reviewed. This evidence was relevant to babies living in all countries and in all conditions.

The recommendations may change again. More evidence is always needed. But right now 'around six months' seems right.

There are different ways to feed a baby solid food. Broccoli can be held by its convenient little handle and baby gums can mash down and take mouthfuls of stuff directly from the source. Or it can be steamed and pureed and spoon fed. Baby-led weaning is a method where spoon feeding doesn't happen. Baby is in charge. Food is offered in pieces and chunks that can be held in a little baby fist and they just go for it. They sit and feed themselves while you sit and eat your own dinner.

Imagine two families with babies in a restaurant. On one table there is a baby sitting up and in front of him is a selection of finger foods: a bit of pitta bread, some vegetables from mum's plate, some chicken. While his parents eat and talk themselves, he picks up pieces of food and self-feeds. At the other table there is a baby being fed pureed foods. While his parents eat, he sits and watches and perhaps is shown books or toys. When his parents are finished, they ask the restaurant to heat up some puree and then a parent sits and feeds him with a spoon.

Both babies are being fed and getting the nutrition they need. One baby is part of the social experience of the meal and is moving towards feeding independence and one baby isn't quite having the same opportunity.

The advantages of baby-led weaning are that baby is experiencing food as a full sensory world. They touch it, smell it and see its natural colours. They are part of the family meal. Food starts out 'real' and never changes. Some babies may gag when self-feeding finger food but the chances of choking are no more than if a baby was being puree fed. Plus you don't have to worry about eventually transitioning to more solid food. If you are really nervous about choking, this can be a good time to do a course in baby first aid. They are often available cheaply in places like local children's centres or even take some time to look at some videos online: http://www.redcross.org.uk/What-we-do/First-aid/Baby-and-Child-First-Aid/Choking-baby.

You can tell from my description that I'm a fan of baby-led weaning. It's been recently promoted by the work of Gill Rapley, a health visitor who has written some useful books on the process. I heard her speak at a food festival once and she got us to do an exercise. We got into pairs. Someone spoon fed me a puree. I couldn't communicate when I was ready for the next mouthful or easily communicate when I was done. I couldn't smell the food or easily see the colour. The spoons of beige mush kept on coming. It tasted fine but I couldn't even put a hand up to slow the process down or ask for a smell or ask to take a breath. It felt overwhelming and the spoons kept coming. After a few minutes, I started to feel like a torture victim! Clearly I am being melodramatic here but imagine you are breastfed baby who up until now has been fairly in control of their own feeding. Wouldn't it be nice if solid food was an extension of that experience?

Of course, you may feel purees are right for you and be particularly attached to your steamer. Like with most things in parenting, you must do what is right for you. Lots of people combine pureed foods and finger foods in a baby-led weaning style. However I would recommend you at least find out about 'baby-led weaning' as it can be enormous fun.

Food before twelve months is 'just for fun' people sometimes say. Not quite true because in many cases, we will need to give baby additional sources of iron and other micronutrients before twelve months. When babies are born they get stores of iron from you and then as they breastfeed, they receive easily absorbable iron from the breastmilk. There was a time when scientists looked at the iron in breastmilk and thought it looked a bit low but we now know that was misleading as it is absorbed incredibly efficiently and is very bioavailable. Studies have shown that when babies are exclusively breastfed for as long as eight or nine months, they still have sufficient levels of iron in their system. However the recommendation to start solids at around six months gives them plenty of time to get up and running before we need to worry about there being a problem. It simply isn't true that because we are now starting a little later, we're in a huge rush to get huge bowlfuls of food into our baby or the world will end. We have time. It's really important to remember that milk remains the primary source of nutrition up until twelve months. It's only at twelve months that solids starts to take equal status and then gradually becomes to primary source of nutrition. Some eighteen month olds are still happily breastfeeding several times a day (and at night) alongside solids and it's a valuable part of their nutrition. These statistics are helpful: In the second year (twelve to twenty three months), 448 mL of breastmilk provides: 29% of energy requirements, 43% of protein requirements, 36% of calcium requirements, 75% of vitamin A requirements, 76% of folate requirements, 94% of vitamin B12 requirements, 60% of vitamin C requirements (Dewey 2001). That's not me saying everyone should breastfeed for twenty three months. That's me saying breastmilk continues to have good stuff in it, the best stuff. It's not going to turn into some useless white fluid when your baby reaches six months and now it's all about the mashed banana.

Some people are concerned about how they are going to time their solid food meals. They are also worried about how to go about 'dropping' a breastfeed and reduce breastmilk appropriately. This is one of the great things about breastfeeding and introducing solids – you don't have to stress about any of that. It happens naturally and organically and your baby is in charge with very little assistance from us. You just continue to breastfeed to your baby's cues. That's it. Bottlefeeding mums do have to plan things out more carefully. Breastfeeding mums just continue to response to their baby's cues and just ensure that the solids intake doesn't increase too quickly.

When you introduce their first solids, think 'milk first'. That means we don't feed a solid meal when a breastfeed is due and then find they aren't that hungry for breastmilk. Better to offer solid food in between breastfeeds or not long after a breastfeed. Food is like a new activity. You've introduced this wonderful new toy that tastes a lot better than the plastic giraffe they've been chewing on for a while. When two meals start to happen, milk is still 'first'. It doesn't have to be first in the sense that you breastfeed and then run from the sofa and plunge them into their high chair – just not long after or a few hours after. We don't want the quantities of breastmilk they receive to really change much for a while. As they start to take more solids, gradually over a 24 hour period, they will take less breastmilk. You may not even notice it happening. Feeds may become a little shorter and intervals between breastfeeds a little longer. It will happen very naturally.

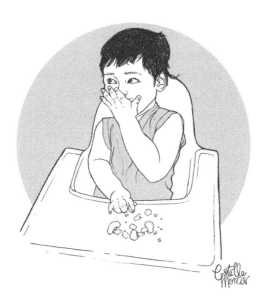

Going Back to Work

The first few weeks are often a blur for new mums. If you remember to shower and put food in the fridge for yourself, you are lucky. For those in the middle of that blur, the thought of the eventual return to work can be one that provokes anxiety.

You can't imagine how it will feel to leave this new special person in your life.

What do you do if you don't want to give up breastfeeding?

Here are my SIX top tips for returning to work as a breastfeeding mum.

1. Don't think about it.

   Ok, now I don't mean that too literally. My message is just that if you are going to take six months, eight months or a year off work and you spend several months of that stressing about the return to work, you will be seriously missing out.

   STOP yourself thinking about it too much. If you stare at your gorgeous three month old and think fleetingly, "How can I ever leave you?" (which is how nature very much wants you to feel), that is fair enough. But if you spend chunks of your maternity leave feeling anxious and worrying about practicalities, you will be wasting the special times you do have together.

This time is precious. Your baby now is not going to be the same person when you return back to work. They will sleep differently, feed differently, and interact differently. You will not be leaving THIS baby but an older one. So get your childcare sorted (which you may well have thought about in pregnancy anyway) and other than that, there's not too much more to do! If you intend to express milk at work, it's a good idea to write to your employer about two months before you go back to work to talk about arrangements. And then just carry on as normal. If your four month old baby won't take a bottle and that starts you panicking because you have to go back to work at eight months, don't think about it. An eight month old baby can breastfeed when you are with them in the morning and evening, take a sippy cup, drink from an open cup – you will have options. And a four month old baby that refuses a bottle may not if you try again after leaving it for a few weeks. It's very easy to set yourself into a panic when the truth is that things usually work out with the right information and the right support.

2. As mentioned, speak to your employer.
    http://www.hse.gov.uk/mothers/faqs.htm#q14
    http://www.nhs.uk/Conditions/pregnancy-and-baby/
    Pages/breastfeeding-back-to-work.aspx

    The recommendation is that you inform them

that you will be returning to work as breastfeeding mum so they have a chance to assess your health and safety and what provisions you may need. Your employers are required to keep you safe. They also have a legal requirement to allow you to 'rest' as a breastfeeding mother. Sadly, in the UK, there is not an explicit legal right to express breastmilk at work but it could be implied if you look at the health and safety requirements employers must meet. It's important you talk to your employer so they have advanced warning and you can come to an arrangement. Some women need to have break times reorganised or a room found. Although there is no spelt-out legal right the VAST majority of employers understand that it is in their interests to try and meet your needs and provide you with facilities. It is possible that they would be vulnerable to a claim of discrimination if they were to refuse you. Hopefully it won't need to get to that stage. Your morale matters and a baby receiving breastmilk is less likely to suffer from illness meaning less time off work for you. There are health and safety executive recommendations and many employers understand the benefits of supporting you as much as possible. However, employers will be more likely to be accommodating if you give them warning and explain your needs clearly.

3. Talk through your schedule with a breastfeeding counsellor or lactation consultant.

Drop-ins are not just for people with problems with positioning and attachment. It's really common for a mum to come along a few weeks before their return to work to talk about how they hope to organise their feeding and pumping schedule and how to organise things practically. I've included some typical scenarios later on.

4. Practise pumping.

Is the breast pump you are using a home something you are familiar with? Do you have a backup if you need to pump at work? Is it worth sourcing a double pump if time is an issue or even hiring a hospital grade electric breast pump for a few months which can just stay at work? You'd be looking at paying around £45 a month (http://www.ardobreastpumps.co.uk/breastpumps_for_hire)

There are tricks such as preparing the breast using massage and warm compresses. And we know that women who finish a pumping session using hand expression techniques can increase their output considerably.

Search for "Stanford University Maximising Milk Production" for some tips.

It's also not a bad idea to build up a bit of a freezer stash before you go back. If you start pumping for one extra session each day and storing that in a freezer bag (store them flat and build up layers of thin flat bags which defrost more easily and take up less space), you will have some wiggle room if you need it. It's not entirely predictable how pumping will go at work and some women find that their pumping output decreases towards the end of the week and then a weekend of normal breastfeeding boosts it back up again. If you have that freezer stash, it will take away some of their anxiety.

5. Get your kit.

    So you need a pump and some bottles and some breastmilk storage bags. What else? Surprisingly not much. You don't need to store freshly expressed breastmilk in the fridge at work if you don't want to. You can have a freezer block and an insulated bag and put any expressed milk in there. It is fine in that for 24 hours. So if you store it like that at work, put it in the fridge when you get home, then that milk can be given to your baby's carer for the next day.
    http://www.breastfeedingnetwork.org.uk/pdfs/ BFNExpressing&Storing.pdf

    It's also really important to note you don't need to wash and sterilise the pump between pumping sessions. Breastmilk is fine at room temperature for up to six hours. So you certainly don't need to wash a pump between your 11am pumping session and your 2pm one. Lots of working mums use a technique called 'wet-bagging', putting a pump in a plastic bag between sessions and then putting it back in the fridge. Then simply take it out next time and wipe any wet parts with paper kitchen towel if you don't fancy cold drips against you! This also saves precious time.

6. Breastfeed when you can.
    Your supply is more likely to be maintained if you breastfeed when you get the chance. Is your childcare near work or home? Could you visit your baby at lunchtime? Could you work from home for one day a week for the first few weeks? You could breastfeed early in the morning, then once more at drop-off, once more at pick-up and again at home later in the evening. Those four feeds would be enough breastmilk overall for a baby of eight months or more. You may not need to be carrying bottles back and forth. And breastfeeding at the weekends and during holidays will help to boost your supply.

Here's Carla's story:
    Carla is going back to work full-time at six months. When her son is four months old, she writes to her boss (she is a PA in a law firm) and explains she is going to continue breastfeeding and wants to express. Her boss explains they have a small room set aside for pumping with a fridge available. Carla plans to express around three times in the working day, once in her lunch break. She has a double electric pump which she starts using from four months and she gives her son a bottle every other day to get him used to it.
    She starts solids around ten days before she goes back

to work. He has two trial days at nursery where Carla practices her expressing schedule and the nursery workers give him a bottle and some solids.

On her working day, she breastfeeds at around 6am. She drops him off at nursery at 7.45am and he takes a small feed. At work she expresses at 11am, 1.30pm and 3.30pm. She collects her son from nursery at 6pm and they breastfeed there. She breastfeeds him again at home at around 10pm as a dreamfeed. He wakes once for another feed at around 2am.

While he is at nursery, the carers give him bottles and offer solids and he usually takes around 12oz. Carla expresses more milk at work than her son takes in a bottle at the moment. Over the next few weeks, she moves to expressing only twice. Carla ends up offering exclusive breastmilk until twelve months and then she gradually introduces cow's milk.

Phoebe is returning to work at ten months. She is a graphic designer and works from home with some client visits necessary around London. Her daughter breastfeeds around four times in 24 hours and enjoys solids which she started at six months. Phoebe doesn't enjoy pumping and finds it difficult so would rather avoid it if possible. She finds a child-minder who lives near her home. Phoebe breastfeeds at 8.30am and drops her daughter at the child-minder. If she is working from home she visits at lunchtime for another breastfeed. She then collects her daughter at around 4pm and takes her home to breastfeed at 6pm and around 11pm. While her daughter is at the child-minder, she eats solid food and drinks water. The child-minder doesn't give her milk. When Phoebe has a client visit, she sometimes hand expresses for a few minutes into a plastic bag when she can grab a private moment. This is just to stay comfortable when she feels particularly engorged. This will help to reduce her risk of blocked ducts and mastitis and help to maintain her supply. She doesn't keep the milk. Phoebe continues breastfeeding her daughter until she is eighteen months old. At the end she is only breastfeeding in the morning and evening and Phoebe doesn't feel the need to use any hand expression when they are separated.

Catherine is returning to work at eight months. Her son breastfeeds around six times in 24 hours. He started solids at six months. He doesn't particularly like bottles and usually only takes around 2oz max. Catherine finds that he will take more milk from an open cup called a doidy cup. He will also more likely to take it if she mixes the breastmilk with ripe banana and makes a smoothie! Catherine gets through a lot of bananas! She works four days a week (and at twelve months will go back to being full time). Catherine is a teacher. Her headteacher has struggled to find her a private room for pumping but has given her the key to the medical room and if that is in use, she uses a stock cupboard and she has told staff that when her scarf is on the door, please knock! Usually the medical room is empty. Her colleagues have agreed to relieve her of playground duty while she is breastfeeding. She breastfeeds her son at 5.45am and again at 7.45am at the child-minder. She arrives at school at 8.15am. She expresses at 10.45am during morning break. She expresses for ten minutes. She expresses again at lunchtime for fifteen minutes and at around 4pm for another ten minutes. She has to use a double pump as her pumping time is restricted. She remains at school for meetings and lesson preparation and collects her son at around 6pm. She breastfeeds him at 7pm and 10pm. He wakes to feed between 1-2am and Catherine is happy for that to continue for the time being as he feeds and goes back to sleep quickly.

With the child-minder, her son takes around 3oz of breastmilk in his smoothie, 2oz mixed into a porridge and another 1-2oz from his doidy cup. She also makes sure his solids contain good sources of fats and calcium. Sometimes she struggles to pump in her breaks as she really needs to continue working. She finds herself dipping into her freezer stash and as time goes on, the child-minder sometimes uses formula to make up the porridge. On the weekends and on her day off, he breastfeeds more frequently.

There are many women who effortlessly combine breastfeeding and working. If it sounds hard, remember that in the USA there is no statutory maternity leave and women often return to work after just a few weeks. However they have 16% of babies exclusively receiving breastmilk at six months and the UK manages 1% (http://www.cdc.gov/breastfeeding/pdf/2012BreastfeedingReportCard.pdf).

With modern electric breast pumps and using breastfeeding support available locally and through helplines, it's never been easier to combine work and breastfeeding. Drop in to a local breastfeeding support group and talk through your plans.

Ending Breastfeeding

In the UK, the recommendation from the Department of Health is to exclusively breastfeed for six months and then introduce solid food. Then to continue to breastfeed alongside solid food for as long as mother and baby wish.

The World Health Organisation say that the ideal length of time to breastfeed is "two years and beyond". This recommendation applies to those living in developed countries as well as the developing world and is based around research on a young child's developing immune system.

If the idea of 'two years and beyond' makes your hair stand on end, you don't need to think about it now. It's hard to imagine what your baby will look like in a month, let alone in a year. Take each day and each week as it comes and just see how you feel. No one is going to sign you up on a list or produce a written contract to become 'an extended breastfeeder'.

Most people that go a bit longer didn't plan on starting out that way. Time just potters by. Breastfeeding is working for them. Everyone finds it a lovely and useful part of the routine and there seems no reason to end it.

Some people go on to practise what's known as 'child-led weaning'. The nursling gradually decides when it's time to stop. It happens slowly (very rarely abruptly – that's probably what's known as a 'nursing strike') and gently and peacefully. Towards the end, an older child might only be breastfeeding once a day and then skip a few days and ask again.

Other people practise 'mother-led weaning'. They start to drop breastfeeds and under twelve months they will need to replace them with bottles of formula milk.

A lot of people operate on a spectrum where the breastfeeding relationship ends with a bit of give and take on both sides.

You don't need to decide in advance.

If your nursling is over twelve months, you can move them straight on to drinking full-fat cow's milk. There's no need to buy any special milks made by formula companies with toddlers in mind. There's a lot of marketing aimed at making you think otherwise but it really isn't needed and many of the added ingredients are unnecessary. You also don't need to introduce bottles to an older baby. The recommendation is to wean off bottles by twelve months so if a baby is older than six months, you may just want to start them off on sippy cups or an open cup.

If your nursling is very attached to using the breast to get themselves to sleep, it's probably worth addressing that before you start to wean. Imagine you'd always fallen asleep a certain way, one that was peaceful and cosy and loving, and then suddenly it was announced you had to fall asleep with a completely different method. That might take some getting used to.

This does NOT mean that you should avoid letting your newborn fall asleep on the breast in preparation for the day you'll eventually want to wean. Falling asleep on the breast is very natural. There are sedatives in breastmilk which are there to encourage it to happen.

However if your toddler is still doing it and you now want to end breastfeeding, let's help them out and give them some new sleeping skills first. A really good resource is 'The No-Cry Sleep Solution' by Elizabeth Pantley. She has a book for babies and one for toddlers and pre-schoolers. She talks you through how to establish a different way of helping them to fall asleep and talks you through her 'pull-off' technique.

When weaning an older child, don't think, "Substitute each breastfeeding with a bottle or cup of milk." Breastfeeding is about connection and emotion as well as nutrition. If they've asked for a breastfeed and are presented with a cup of milk, it's an odd response. Get the nutrients they need into them at some point over 24 hours and have lots of cuddles. Someone once told me reading books together is a more appropriate substitute for a breastfeed than a cup of cow's milk. I can see their point.

Try and avoid being asked in the first place so you never get to the point of rejection. One method of weaning is known as 'Don't offer, Don't refuse'. Use distraction. Mix up the routine. Scoop them up and do a silly dance if they get an 'asking' glint in their eye.

With a younger baby, you are dropping a feed every

three to four days and substituting it with a bottle. You take a few days before dropping a breastfeed to give your breasts a chance to adjust and reduce your supply.

If you move too quickly, you may find yourself suffering from engorgement and even blocked ducts that could lead to mastitis.

If you do feel really uncomfortable between feeds, you may express off just a tiny amount of milk but obviously during this process, we need to tell the body to make less milk and being engorged is how that process happens.

After breastfeeding has ended, some people do still feel a bit sore. It can be helpful to eat dry or fresh sage to reduce milk supply. Cool compresses or cabbage leaves can also be useful.

It's not unusual for mums to find themselves having an emotional reaction to the ending of breastfeeding. We've losing all that lovely oxytocin so YOU need lots of cuddles and contact as much as baby does.

Tidbits

What follows are mini-chapters on a variety of different topics that don't fit neatly into a concept of chronology. You might be struggling with sore nipples on day three or month three.

Finding Help in the UK

Breastfeeding support in the UK can be a bit of a postcode lottery. It's a good idea to research what's available in your area when you are pregnant. Ask your midwife which of the four breastfeeding charities are active. Find the breastfeeding counsellors and peer supporters. Find the lactation consultants. Accessing a private lactation consultant isn't an option available to everyone for financial reasons. You may be paying £50-£100 for a session with a lactation consultant in your home depending on where you live. It's actually a weird profession where we wish we didn't have to exist. In Utopia, there would be no private lactation consultants in the UK. Your midwife would be educated to a lactation consultant standard. Your health visitor would be. And why not? What could be more important than how you FEED the baby? You can find a lactation consultant by searching on www.lcgb.org.

Isn't a bit daft that peer supporters provide the breastfeeding support in some areas? Imagine if you suffered from migraines to the extent you could barely function and you were in agony and the NHS's response was to put you in touch with a very nice lady who'd had migraines for a while. You'd think, "Sod off! I need someone who has all the knowledge at their finger tips and has the time to devote to this. Someone who is fully trained. The system should get how important this is." That is sort of true. Instead think of peer supporters as a community of useful women rather than the 'experts'. In that expression, 'it takes a village to raise a child', they are part of that village. We need them because we may not have friends who breastfed or live near our breastfeeding sisters and cousins. When things get more complicated, you may need to go further so good peer supporters will always be able to signpost you onto breastfeeding counsellors and lactation consultants and feeding specialists who know more.

In the UK, a health visitor or midwife may have the same level of knowledge as a peer supporter. Or they may have the same level of knowledge as a lactation consultant. There's a huge variation. You may have a golden health visitor who is a key person in your breastfeeding success and is someone you will always look back on with fondness and gratitude. You may have a health visitor who seemed a bit confused about some of the breastfeeding basics and you needed to find answers elsewhere.

The helplines are a good source of support in the UK. The National Breastfeeding Helpline is staffed from volunteers from the Association of Breastfeeding Mothers and the Breastfeeding Network. http://nationalbreastfeedinghelpline.org.uk/. The number is 0300 100 0212. It is open from 9.30am to 9.30pm 365 days a year.

These charities also have their own helplines (from the NHS website):

- Association of Breastfeeding Mothers is a charity run by mothers for mothers, giving friendly support and supplying accurate information to all women wanting to breastfeed. We also have an email counselling service. www.abm.me.uk. Helpline number: 0300 330 5453. The helpline is open from 9.30 am to 10.30 pm.
- Breastfeeding Network provides breastfeeding support and information for mothers and those involved in their care. Helpline number: 0300 100 0210.
- The NCT is a leading charity for parents, supporting people through pregnancy, birth and early parenthood. Helpline: 0300 330 0771 8am to midnight. http://www.nct.org.uk/about-nct/contact-us/one-one-support
- We also have the La Leche League GB who have a network of local groups and a helpline open 8am to 11pm: Telephone Helpline 0845 120 2918

With the exception of the NCT (who pay some of their BFCs), the helplines are staffed by volunteers in their own homes. It takes about two years to train to be a breastfeeding counsellor (while a peer supporter course usually takes a couple of hours a week for ten weeks). A La Leche League leader, ABM breastfeeding counsellor, NCT breastfeeding counsellor and Breastfeeding Network supporter are all equivalent qualifications and the training is evidence-based. You should end up getting the same answer from all of these helplines and the information they give will be based on research and not opinion.

If you have a question about whether you can breastfeed while taking a certain medication, you can contact the 'drugs in breastmilk' service. Their contact details are here along with some factsheets which may provide the answer without you needing to contact them: http://www.breastfeedingnetwork.org.uk/detailed-information/ drugs-in-breastmilk/

Complications: My Baby Won't Attach

When you were preparing for this breastfeeding thing, you were worried it might hurt. Your sister-in-law worried you that your baby might feed 'all the time'. You were concerned how you were going to breastfeed in public.

Now you wish you were so lucky to have a baby that 'fed all the time'. If only you could experience breastfeeding at ALL, even if it hurt a bit. You envy the women who have a problem feeding in Starbucks. You should be so lucky.

Breast refusal is scary. It wasn't what you were expecting. You thought this little person would come out wanting to do it. No one told you anything else was possible. Your antenatal class teacher showed you some amazing video of a baby crawling up their post-birth mummy's body and self-attaching. Trouble is – it seems your own baby hasn't seen the same videos.

The 2010 infant feeding survey says that 27% of mothers stop breastfeeding in the first week because their baby was completely rejecting the breast or not latching properly. There are lots of people struggling with this problem and a lot of breastfeeding counsellors and lactation consultants trying to help them.

Just to say, it is completely normal for babies to sometimes appear to reject the breast in the course of normal successful breastfeeding. Just like we sometimes don't fancy a meal, babies are the same. They don't care what the clock says. Sometimes they are simply too tired or over-stimulated. Perhaps they are dealing with something to do with lower digestion and a pool is imminent. Sometimes they have some upper wind and although they are apparently hungry, it seems like some mysterious force field is preventing them from latching on. These are babies that may take a few hours before they feed successfully again but they will usually get there in the end. If we are seeing wet nappies, periods of alertness and there are no other medical concerns, we may just have to wait a while. We continue to skin-to-skin. We try different positions. It happens in the end.

Newborn breast refusal is a different thing. Sometimes these are babies who did manage to feed a handful of times over a few days but we are usually talking about babies who have yet to latch on successfully and transfer milk. They may refuse to latch at all and bob on the breast in a frustrated and desperate way. They may appear to latch with the right gape and positioning. It actually does look like those photos from your antenatal class, but when the baby is 'on' nothing seems to actually happen. It is like the photo – immobile and not the video version. They just sit there and fall asleep quite quickly.

What are we going to do? Here are the first four rules when a newborn baby isn't breastfeeding (credit to IBCLC Linda Smith for the last three).

1. Don't panic.

I know that sounds trite but new mums are awash with hormones and especially if your birth wasn't what you expected, a non-attaching baby can be a very frightening concept. You really weren't prepared for this. Does this mean you are never going to breastfeed?

It is very, very, very important to hear this next part: with the right information and support, most mums of non-attaching babies will be able to breastfeed after a short while. There is a small minority for whom there are further complications but this is a minority. I have known many, many mums (and I was one of them) who had a baby who didn't attach properly for the first few days and went on to breastfeed happily for as long as they wanted to, for months and even years.

I rarely share my own breastfeeding experience but Sam's story is relevant here. When I was giving birth to Sam in 2004, my labour moved very quickly for a first baby. When I was in transition and felt ready to push, I called the midwife in and she shook her head with a smile and said, "Honey, no. You've got hours and hours to go yet. This is still early days." This was without any examination or having been in the room with me any time recently. It was a back-to-back labour which can be quite uncomfortable and my birth plan suddenly went out the window. I panicked. She offered me pethidine – an opiate drug. I took it. She explained that it was never sensible to give it just before delivery as it can affect baby but this would be OK as I had 'so long' to go. Sam was born less than half an hour later.

He was OK but he very, very sleepy and although we had a bit of skin-to-skin (which I don't remember being called that then); he really wasn't up to breastfeeding. Luckily another midwife saw the situation and told me to get pumping and syringe feeding. He only breastfed properly for the first time on about day three. He was initially syringe-fed colostrum and never needed any other milk.

Sometimes non-attachment is about the birth experience. Drugs that relieve our pain can annoyingly affect baby too. The first breastfeed and the first few days can be a far greater challenge when we're waiting for things to get back to normal. Research is very clear that even drugs seen as less hard core than pethidine, like in an epidural, impact on early breastfeeding success over the first 24 hours: (http://www.ncbi.nlm.nih. gov/pubmed/12583645) And we can get into a cascade where a mum doesn't get those early feeds to happen, is encouraged to use a bottle or supplement in another way and she's then not dealing with the consequences of the epidural but the decisions that led from that. Some babies born with forceps or ventouse can experience cranial nerve bruising and discomfort which make the mechanics of early breastfeeding a struggle. Unfortunately the baby is unable to convey the fact they have experienced compression of the glossopharyngeal, hypoglossal or vagus nerve so please give them a while. If you have a headache, imagine the act of opening your mouth really really wide or someone holding the side of your head.

Are we saying that all babies who have assisted deliveries or whose mums take pain relief will struggle? No, of course not. Many will be fine and breastfeed well but this is about likelihood. I don't know anyone who has turned down a forceps delivery when it's recommended to them and that's not what this is about. It's about having information. Talk to your doctor when induction is suggested a week after the due date. What's the evidence base for that decision because that may increase the chance of pain relief or an assisted delivery and that may make breastfeeding more of a challenge? If you are going down a certain road, know that breastfeeding support may be more of a priority. You may need to place an even higher emphasis on skin-to-skin after birth (though I hope it was high on your list anyway) and you may need a breast pump.

But we're still not panicking because even if things go initially a bit pear-shaped, it's likely you can still make breastfeeding happen. You follow these rules. You talk to people around you who know about breastfeeding. You look after yourself. You say hello to your gorgeous new baby who isn't doing this on purpose and would really like to breastfeed too.

2. Rule two is feed the baby. I know that might sound obvious but you'd be surprised. I've known situations where trying to breastfeed takes ages and ages and baby and mum and everyone are tired and baby drifts off to sleep and no actual milk was transferred. Then baby wakes up and there's another attempt to breastfeed. Sleepy young babies then start to conserve energy and sleep more (which makes breastfeeding even less likely). If we're going to work on this, we need some fuel. Plus we obviously want baby to be hydrated and not lose too much weight – though it's important to note that baby's aren't expected to take in a lot of milk in the first couple of days and are expected to lose some weight. We don't need to glug huge quantities into them. Early feeds are teaspoons worth. However they get the gut moving, get the poo happening and have a PhD's worth of useful purposes.

Hopefully if baby isn't breastfeeding, you are being shown how to take the milk out of your breasts immediately. There's a nice video on breast massage and hand expression here: http://bfmedneo.com/

This is a time when the mums who did some hand expression antenatally are at an advantage. You can read more about that option here: http://abm.me.uk/expressing-milk-baby-arrives-antenatal-expression-colostrum/

You can collect the colostrum in a syringe and ask someone to show you how to give it to baby using a cup or a syringe. I like syringe feeding as it means there is nothing wasted and you can pop your finger against the roof of baby's mouth and get some sucking happening with the tongue extended over the gum ridge and a rhythm developing. Baby isn't flat on their back but elevated enough to reduce the risk of aspiration. Baby starts to suck on your clean finger and you reward with a little bit of milk from the syringe in the corner of their mouth. Cup feeding also gets the tongue extended but it's usually something you need to be taught.

Bottle-feeding isn't considered first choice because it can teach incorrect tongue positioning, poor gaping and milk will flow without baby needing to use their muscles in the normal way. However if it's day three and baby hasn't fed for eight hours and you are panicking and you can't get hold of the midwife, giving a bottle may be a more sensible choice than not. You're just going to try and do in a way that is as close to breastfeeding as possible. Have a look on YouTube for some videos on 'paced bottle-feeding'. Some are quite extreme but take the principle that we want the baby to create negative space in their mouth and remove milk with effort. If the bottle is more horizontal and the baby is more upright, that is more likely to happen. The milk should not be so fast that the baby is overwhelmed and they are struggling to maintain breathing. Bottle feeding babies have lower oxygenation rates when they are feeding anyway so let's be extra careful with flow.

We also want a baby feeding on the bottle to have a mouth that looks like a baby feeding on the breast. It seems logical to still hope that the baby will gape with a wide mouth. When they breastfeed, they fill their oral cavity with stuff. It seems sensible to do the same thing when we bottle-feed rather than have a baby nipple-feeding with pursed lips. Let's put the nipple to the top lip, 'nose to nipple'. When the baby gapes we will bring the bottle into baby's mouth when it is still wide. If the baby's bottom lip is flanged down, that's a good sign that the tongue is extending over the gum ridge rather than being pushed back as it can with artificial nipples. It may be more difficult to get a baby to do anything other than nipple-feed on bottles that have long nipples and very little areola/ breast behind them. And a word of warning, it's amazing how many bottles seem to be the 'closest to the breast'. It's never going to be close and it's going to depend which bit of the experience of breastfeeding you are prioritising. If we used paced bottle-feeding, we can slow the flow so I think it seems wise to try and get a space that allows gaping alongside that.

3. Protect the Milk supply.

So baby is being fed and at number three, we are protecting the milk supply. That's still ahead of trying to breastfeed and practising breastfeeding. If we maintain and protect milk supply, we'll have options once underlying problems have resolved. If we don't, when baby does start feeding it may not last long if they don't find time at the breast rewarding. In the first few weeks, our breast tissue is developing and we are laying down the ground work for our supply that will govern the rest of the time we breastfeed. Stimulating supply now will make difference months down the line. Plus if we don't protect milk supply, we're more likely to get blocked ducts, mastitis, engorgement and abscesses.

A lot of people will tell you that colostrum can only be hand expressed. Colostrum is sticky and there isn't much of it and it can get lost in pumps and flanges. With hand expression, you can gather every drop. However once a day has passed, you may find it useful to start pumping too. It will save time and help your supply really kick in. You could perhaps hand express first and then pump for five to ten minutes. As your milk transitions to mature milk, you may find it's more time efficient to keep going with just the pumping. Some mums find hand expression super easy and continue with that but hand expressing eight to ten times in 24 hours can be hard work.

You can hire hospital grade double electric pumps. Your local NCT branch may have a pump agent. You can also hire direct from ardobreastpumps.co.uk. Pumping shouldn't hurt and take a moment to check you have the right funnel/ flange size. Your pump rental agent can send out alternatives.

When a baby is non-attaching, a typical routine may look like this:

Skin-to-skin, try breastfeeding for fifteen to twenty minutes (if it works and milk is being transferred, go longer!); someone else gives a top-up while mums pumps. Everyone naps.

Repeat.

Ideally you are one ahead on the pumping. That means you don't pump while a hungry baby is waiting for your milk. That's likely to affect the way the milk flows and won't help anyone. You should be pumping for the feed that comes after. Mums often get better pumping results with a bit of breast preparation. Start with breast massage and warm compressions. In research, mums also got a good deal more out when they did some hand expression after the flow from pumping had stopped. Newborn babies cluster feed so you could cluster pump too. Have an hour or so, perhaps in the evening, when you pump for ten minutes, pause for five, pump for ten minutes, pause for five, repeat.

4. Work on the Breastfeeding

When baby is being fed and your supply is being protected, you can work on the breastfeeding.

Skin-to-skin is super important (have I mentioned

that already?). We try to breastfeed when babies are quietly alert or a bit sleepy or hungry or not very hungry or not very hungry at all. You can try after a little bit from the bottle. Don't think the breast always HAS to be first and if you're giving up on the breast, that's it. You could give 10ml from a syringe, try some breastfeeding, a bit more from a syringe, trickle the syringe over the nipple to encourage some licking and rooting. Move between breast and non-breast organically.

All feeds happen at a naked breast.

Try different positions. Have a look at www. biologicalnurturing.com and try some laid back breastfeeding. See if you can encourage some self-attachment.

How do you know milk is being transferred? You may hear some swallowing but not always. You should notice baby's chin moving and occasionally pausing to show a swallow. Dr Jack Newman has a video called 'really good drinking' that may help: http://www.breastfeedinginc.ca/content.php?pagename=vid-reallygood

If you have very flat or inverted nipples, it may appear that baby is searching for something but not quite able to get purchase and stay on. You may need some help learning how to shape your breast and nipple. You may even end up using nipple shields to help a non-attaching baby attach. Nipple shields get a bad rep but this is a situation where they can be useful and a baby may end up breastfeeding as a result. It's always better though to use a shield with some qualified support. They can cause further problems if the wrong sized shield is used, if they are applied poorly and the latch is still a problem.

Getting qualified support is a good idea whatever your nipple look like. You can ask your midwife for local recommendations. Perhaps that person is your midwife or her colleague. You may have a local volunteer breastfeeding counsellor who can meet you at home or who runs a local group. You may choose to pay for a private lactation consultant and you can find one at www. lcgb.org.

It's also sensible to get someone to look inside baby's mouth, someone who knows that tongue tie can affect breastfeeding. I know that might sound daft but some healthcare professionals are poorly trained in tongue tie and it's a leading cause of non-attachment in young babies.

You can read more about tongue tie here: http://www. cwgenna.com/ttidentify.html

Babies can also struggle if they have high palates and this often goes alongside having a tongue tie.

If your baby does have a tongue tie that still doesn't mean you won't be successfully breastfeeding soon. You can learn different positions and breast shaping techniques that can help. Your baby may also benefit from a simple procedure where the membrane that holds their tongue tie is cut with a pair of round-ended scissors. This is called a frenectomy. Your midwife or GP should be able to refer you to your local NHS tongue tie service. You can also find private practitioners here: www.tongue-tie.org.uk.

I know this is scary but please believe that if you find the people that can help you this is still likely to work out.

I know mums who have had a baby finally attached at 48 hours, one week, two weeks, three weeks and six weeks. The 27% who gave up in the first week according to the infant feeding survey weren't speaking to the right people. We were visited at the ABM conference by a mum who attached for the first time at 18 months (that got your attention, didn't it.) No one can tell you how long to keep going with this but it's true that you might give up when there's still a chance your baby will happily attach. You have to decide when it's right for you.

You could certainly continue exclusively breast milk feeding your baby if that's what you want to do. I could write another 3000 words on why that's a good idea. You can read more about exclusive pumping in a useful book written by Stephanie Casemore: http://www.exclusivelypumping.com/

Good luck. Be strong. Find helpers… and did I mention skin-to-skin?

Is your baby older and was previously successfully breastfeeding?

Some babies may start to refuse the breast after a period of successful breastfeeding. That can also be confusing and upsetting. It can happen as a result of flow confusion if they have had regular experience of bottles. In that situation, you could perhaps speed up the flow at the breast (perhaps by increasing supply or using breast compressions). If you've been using bottles a fair bit, your supply may have taken a dip and may need a bit of attention. Breast compressions are useful when the milk starts to get fattier and slower and baby may be finding it a bit harder work. A bit more on breast compressions here: https://www.youtube.com/watch?v=Oh-nnTps1Ls

You can also slow things on the bottle in comparison. The section above on paced bottle-feeding talk you through some of that. If you are confused and unsure, visit your local breastfeeding support group. Don't think they are just for people with new babies and people who don't use bottles.

Breastfeeding babies who've never had a bottle in their lives can also go on nursing strikes. A self-weaning baby doesn't give up breastfeeding overnight; it's normally a gradual and gentle process that takes no one by surprise. It also rarely happens under eighteen months old.

Some good thoughts on nursing strikes here: http://www.lalecheleague.org/faq/strike.html

Get your GP to check baby doesn't have an ear infection and check in baby's mouth. Could your baby have a blocked nose? Most nursing strikes will resolve within a few days. Feed the baby and protect your supply.

Complications: Engorgement

There are two kinds of engorgement. About two to five days after birth, we get what's sometimes known as your 'milk coming in'. This is actually a bit of a misleading term. Your milk has been gradually transitioning ever since the placenta was delivered and the body lost its progesterone factory. It's not as though a switch is flicked on day two. Your breast is becoming filled with lymph fluid and blood surrounding the developing breast tissue. There is milk in there but a lot of that firmness isn't milk inside your glandular tissue but lymph fluid everywhere! Engorgement can vary. For some people with very awake and frequently feeding babies, it's not that noticeable – perhaps a bit of heaviness and discomfort but not hugely so. If baby is sleepy and reluctant to feed or if latching isn't quite sorted, things might be more uncomfortable. It's a good reason to encourage babies to drain the breasts as frequently as you can persuade them to.

When breasts get fuller and tighter, sometimes that means the nipple and areola changes shape too. It can be a bit like baby trying to latch onto a beach ball. Remember apple bobbing? If the skin is very tight, it may not be easy for baby to get a mouthful of breast. Or if they do, they may not have the nipple as far back as is ideal and it might hurt a bit more. That's one reason it's good to practice as much as you can in the first few days so when engorgement does arrive, you already feel pretty confident about the latching process.

126

It can help to express a little bit before a feed to help soften the breast and give baby a bit more to hold onto. Sometimes we may find engorgement makes it difficult for milk to actually flow. The ducts may not have the space they need to do the milk ejection reflex properly and expand. You can experiment with warm compresses. If that doesn't work, you can go in a completely different direction and experiment with cold compresses. This will help to get lymph fluid moving. You can use some frozen peas wrapped in a towel carefully for a few minutes at a time. You can also massage your breasts towards the armpit to get lymph moving. You can also have a go at a technique called 'Reverse Pressure Softening'. This is when you indent your fingers into the areola like the petals around the centre of a flower. You press them there for a few minutes and when you remove your fingers, you should find you've pushed the fluid away from your areola and your nipple area is easier for baby to grasp onto.

Ibuprofen is an anti-inflammatory medication which can be helpful with engorgement and help relieve some of the discomfort. If it was safe for you to take ibuprofen before pregnancy, it's compatible with your breastfeeding.

Some people advocate wearing cabbage leaves. We need to be a bit careful with this as there is some link between cabbage leaves and supply reduction. They are particularly useful when mums are weaning and trying to 'dry up'. It might be better to use a cool gel pack instead if you like the relief of coolness. Breasts can feel quite hot during engorgement by the way.

Hopefully you'll only be uncomfortable for a couple of days.

If you end up feeling engorged later on in your breastfeeding experience it might mean something is shifting. Perhaps baby is starting to sleep longer at night and your breasts wake up before baby does. Perhaps baby is starting to naturally extend their intervals between feeds and you are feeling fuller (which then adjusts your supply a little). However we generally want to avoid being engorged if we can. It can sometimes mean something isn't quite right with positioning and attachment and perhaps the breast isn't being drained as efficiently as it should be. It increases your chances of blocked ducts and mastitis. It is also likely to reduce supply. It is also more likely to make latching tricky. Don't ever assume that feeling engorged is the goal because it means there's lots of milk there and think you should 'wait to feel full'. Once milk has transitioned to mature milk and you're breastfeeding effectively and in response to baby's cues you may hardly ever get engorged again.

Complications: Blocked Ducts and Mastitis

A relatively high proportion of mums will experience blocked ducts at some point. Some of these mums will end up developing mastitis but you can reduce the risk of this happening by knowing what to do when a blocked ducts appears.

The phrase 'blocked duct' is a bit misleading. It suggests we're just worrying about a blob of something unhelpful stuck inside a tube and if we can just dislodge it, all will be well. What usually happens is that a bit too much milk gets left behind in the breast (there's always some milk left behind but a bit more in this case) and it ends up leaking into tissue where milk is not normally stored. The breast sees the milk as an invading foreign body and sends the immune response – extra lymph fluid and blood. The breast ends up with a firm tender area. It may present as a lump or more like a wedge. If you don't manage to sort things out and keep the breast well-drained, bacteria may arrive in the area. This is when you may notice the breast getting redder and becoming even more tender and you'll start to feel rough and fluey. After 12-24 hours, you would need to visit your GP for some antibiotics.

But hopefully we can avoid that stage by sorting out the blocked ducts in the first place. How do we do that?

It's a good idea to get used to how your breasts feel when they are full and empty. When they feel quite full, you'll notice that you can sometimes feel lumpy bits under the skin. Some mums instantly panic this means blocked ducts but actually you may well be feeling the alveoli, milk storage areas which are like a cluster of grapes. Wait and feel again after the feed. A blocked duct will be hanging around.

If that lump is remaining, we'll need to start by

checking a few things. Is your bra well-fitting? Are you holding your breast while you feed or pressing your finger into your breast because someone told you if you didn't, your baby couldn't breathe <rolling eyes emoticon>? Is your sling pressing into your breast? Or a bag?

How is your positioning and attachment? Any sore or misshapen nipples? If there is a problem with latching, this might mean that an area of your breast isn't being drained properly and consistently a bit too much milk is being left behind.

Some mums who have recurrent blocked ducts find it helpful to take a supplement called lecithin. It's an ingredient used by the food industry in ready meals as it changes the way fat behaves and prevents it sticking together in big globules. The theory is this will then make the fat in your breastmilk a bit smoother running. We don't have reliable evidence on this but if you are suffering regularly and looked at other potential causes, it might be worth looking into.

If part of your breast feels firm and things don't get easier after a feed, we have a window of time to sort things out before mastitis might develop. We need to keep the breast well-drained. This means feeding at least every three hours. If baby doesn't want to feed (and sometimes this might happen when you are away from baby or perhaps baby is reluctant to feed), you'll need to get pumping. Use warm compresses on the breast before you do any draining. You can fill a disposable nappy with hot water and wrap it round the breast or immerse the breast in a bath of hot water. Then try some massage; circular massage on the firm area and also stroking down towards your nipple. You can also use an electric toothbrush to firmly massage on the lump (you can always wrap the end in cling film). Then when it comes time to feed, perhaps vary things by using different positions. You can use a dangle feed, placing baby in the centre of a double bed and literally dangle over them with the breast hanging free. You could also experiment with pointing baby's chin towards the firm area (though this may not always be reliable as milk ducts can wiggle around quite a lot). After a feed, try a bit more massage and warm compresses.

Take a look at the end of your nipple. Is there any sign of a white blister filled with milk known as a bleb? There could be a thin layer of skin over the end of a milk duct preventing the breast draining properly. You can put heat on it and some pressure behind it and you may be able to dislodge it. Or try soaking in a warm salty solution or applying warm olive oil on cotton wool. Sometimes, if it isn't going anywhere, it may be a good idea to pierce it with a sterile needle. You need to be very careful not to cause further damage. You ideally want to nick just the end of it so you can then squeeze out the contents rather than cause some huge hole. Don't push the needle towards your body but pick at it with the sharp end of a needle away from your body, then you won't accidentally push it in too far. Then get feeding and draining the breast as usual.

If that firm area remains for more than 24 hours, if you get a red patch on the breast or a red line, if you start to get a temperature and feel like you have flu, you should make an appointment to see your GP. If you do need antibiotics, still continue with all the other self-help measures like frequent drainage and massage. You should always continue to drain the breast and continue feeding once mastitis has been diagnosed. If you don't, or if you don't finish a course of antibiotics, there's a chance you may develop an abscess where there is pocket of pus in the breast that will need to be removed. That's a hassle that's best avoided.

Complications: Thrush

Thrush (which is a sneaky little fungus called Candida Albicans) likes dark moist environments. Prior to breastfeeding, you may have only been worried about finding it in your underwear but disappointingly thrush likes breasts too. It can also be found in folds of skin on baby and in baby's nappy area which is why good hygiene and good drying after bathing and washing is so important.

When we breastfeed, we tuck a moist nipple back inside a bra which may also have a moist breast pad in it and occasionally that can lead to problems.

Usually our bodies are good at keeping thrush at bay. We live symbiotically with a family of friendly bacteria that help us keep thrush under control. When we have antibiotics (which many mums do at birth or just

*Prior to breastfeeding, you may have
only been worried about finding it in
your underwear but disappointingly
thrush likes breasts too.*

afterwards) or if we have nipple damage or if we get run down, things may get out of balance.

When mums develop thrush on their nipple, they often report the nipple feels much more sensitive and anything brushing against it is excruciating. Nipples can sometimes appear pinker than usual or may have a scaly flaky look about them. Both nipples will be affected as thrush is very transferable. You may notice that baby also has symptoms in their mouth. You can see white blobs that look a bit like cotton wool or cottage cheese on the inside of the cheeks, inside lips or on the roof of the mouth. There might be a pearly sheen inside their lips. Sometimes you may see thickness on the back of the tongue but baby's tongues can also have a milky coating anyway so don't confuse it with that. Also don't confuse it for an Epstein Pearl. This is a teeny little white blob that newborns often have on their hard palate and is nothing to worry about.

Babies may not always have symptoms even if mum does. But if you do have thrush, you will both still need treatment. The Breastfeeding Network is a good source of information on the latest way to treat thrush. Ideally you would have topical anti-fungal cream and baby would have oral gel which also contains the same active ingredient, usually miconazole. Unfortunately the gel isn't licensed for young babies as there was an incident where a smaller baby choked on a blob so nystatin suspension is often given instead. The key thing with any thrush treatment for baby is that you're not trying to get baby to swallow it. It works by coming into contact with surfaces like the inside of the cheeks, roof of the mouth and inside of lips. Try and coat the inside of the mouth and keep it hanging around as long as you can (so don't apply it just before a feed).

When you're fighting thrush, remember that thrush likes a dark moist environment so changing breast pads frequently and some light exposure is a good idea. Some mums find it's helpful to rinse with a solution of vinegar (thrush doesn't like acid) or even use a mixture of vinegar and water to slosh bras in before putting them in the washing machine.

You may also want to take some friendly bacteria (perhaps lacto acidophilus capsules) as it was likely a lack of friendly bacteria that caused a problem in the first place. Grapefruit seed extract is also a fungicide many mums take.

Ductal thrush is something you may hear people talking about. If you have deep breast pain, you will often google and get to people talking about ductal thrush.

However this is a rare cause of deep breast pain and in fact there are some sensible scientists who feel that it's rare to almost the point of being non-existent and cultures of women experiencing deep breast pain are more likely to show a bacterial problem than a fungal one (or have deeper breast pain because of latching issues and problems at the nipple). It's also complicated because the treatment for ductal thrush (a tablet called fluconazole) is not straight forward to prescribe. It's not licensed for breastfeeding mums. Sometimes drugs aren't licensed because the faff of doing proper safety trials is not something pharmaceutical companies are willing to pay for. It's cheaper for them to hope a doctor will take full responsibility. Something not being licensed does not automatically mean a drug is unsafe. In this case however, fluconazole has a long half-life which means it hangs around in the system and particularly can accumulate in the liver of young babies. We're not going to want to give large doses to a mother breastfeeding a young baby unless we're really sure we are dealing with thrush.

There are more likely reasons why a mother can have deeper breast pain. It isn't going to be thrush if only one side if affected for starters. Thrush is more rampant than that. Ductal thrush pain is also consistent after every feed and every pumping session so if pumping is less uncomfortable, that doesn't suggest thrush. It's also unlikely to be thrush if a mum has redness on the skin or a temperature (which suggests a bacterial infection). If a mum has visible nipple damage, then the pain may be due to something called neuralgia. When there is nipple compression and nipple pain, the nerve at the end of the nipple is going to be receiving pain signals. This pain message can travel down the course of the nerve that goes right through the breast to get to the spine. We may feel the pain quite deep in the breast. We can get transferred pain in the breasts sometimes because of back pain too. We need to check a mum isn't hunched over and her back is well-supported.

Complications: Tongue tie

The tongue has the starring role in breastfeeding. A baby lifts and extends their tongue towards the breast and forms a seal. They then move their tongue in wave-like motions from front to back which encourages milk to be removed from the breast by creating negative pressure. As a negative space is formed in the mouth when the tongue drops, milk comes out of the breast to fill that space. Some people imagine that baby's squeeze the breast to remove milk. The tongue does also compress the breast but this isn't the whole story. The creation of the vacuum is the important bit. Underneath our tongues many of us have little membranes that attach the tongue to the base of our mouths. You may see it straining when you lift up your tongue in the mirror. If a baby has a frenulum that is too tight and short or if it is too near the tip of the tongue, the baby may struggle to do the job it needs to do. The baby may end up clamping the breast with its gum ridge (when normally the tongue will be covering the gum ridge as the tongue extends). It may hump the rear of the tongue and move the tongue forward but the tongue then snaps back. Mum's nipple can end up rubbing against the rear of the tongue or rubbing against the baby's hard palate as the breast isn't drawn back far enough.

Nipple damage is one sign that things aren't going right. The nipple may also come out looking squashed or flattened or tapered at the end like an old lipstick. The baby's cheeks may get sucked in when they feed as there isn't enough breast filling their mouth. Baby might feed for a long time or feed very frequently or slip off the breast once they are on. Baby might start to have weight gain problems and if the milk isn't being removed effectively, this might lead to supply problems for mum. Sometimes the baby might have a whitish tongue as the top layer of skin isn't getting rubbed off in the normal way.

It's important to note that not all babies with a tongue tie need to have something done about it.

It's important to note that not all babies with a tongue tie need to have something done about it. A lot depends on mum's nipple and breast shape and what other skills a baby can use to breastfeeding comfortably and effectively. Some babies have a frenulum quite near the tip of the tongue but it's a stretchy one so elevation can still happen.

The NICE (NHS) guidelines support doing a tongue tie release if breastfeeding is being negatively affected. This usually means being referred to a local hospital for a frenectomy where the membrane is snipped using a pair of round-ended scissors. Sometimes a scalpel might be used or even a laser. Sometimes the procedure is done in a home setting by a qualified healthcare practitioner. It sounds daft but check that whoever is doing the procedure is a registered healthcare professional (a doctor, nurse, midwife or dentist) as there isn't proper regulation in this field. You can find private practitioners via the Association of Tongue Tie Practitioners (www.tongue-tie.org.uk) and some families choose to go privately if the NHS services local to them are perhaps over-subscribed and the wait is too long. When a baby is having the frenulum cut they don't need an anaesthetic. We actually want sensation to be unaffected so that feeding can continue immediately afterwards. I've observed the procedure several times and babies seem to object more to being held down than the cut itself.

Having the tongue tie cut isn't always an instant fix. It's a muscle that hasn't been able to do its job for a while. Usually babies are busy exercising their tongues months before they are born so it may take a couple of weeks before feeding improves. Tongue tie babies also often have high arched palates or 'bubble palates'. The roof of their mouth is a high arch, like there was a big marble up there that someone has removed rather than a gentle lit up arched roof of the mouth. This can also make breastfeeding tricky but it should start to drop over the weeks that follow a tongue tie procedure.

Lip tie is something you may hear being discussed especially on social media. There is a lot less evidence supporting the division of a lip tie (a frenulum attaching the lip to the upper gum) and at the moment that means it isn't cut on the NHS to support breastfeeding. Some babies with a posterior tongue tie may also have a lip tie and the posterior tongue tie is being missed and the lip tie is being blamed. There is also a misunderstanding that the baby needs their upper lip to flange right out in a fish lips style like the lower lip does. Actually the upper lip can rest in a neutral position and a very excessive flange can be the sign of a shallow latch. There are rare cases where a very tight and tense upper lip can cause breastfeeding difficulties but it's important to get a proper assessment from someone knowledgeable about breastfeeding first to check that your positioning and attachment is the best it can be and something else more likely isn't being missed.

You sometimes hear people in the breastfeeding support world saying, "There seems to be a lot more tongue tie around than there once was." There are three possibilities: EITHER there are more cases of tongue tie and something is going on with infant anatomy OR there are the same number of cases and we are now seeing more mums wanting to breastfeed and continue breastfeeding OR there are not more cases and babies are being misdiagnosed.

There's a useful guide to tongue tie identification here: http://www.cwgenna.com/ttidentify.html

Complications: Sore Nipples

You may hear people stating that 'breastfeeding should never hurt'. I'm not sure this statement is entirely helpful. In the first few days, your nipple – which up until now has been sitting happily in bras and bikini tops and dealing with only the occasional twiddle – is experiencing some serious stretching. A nipple positioned correctly during breastfeeding is sitting inside a space under negative pressure and being stretched to nearly three times its natural length. It seems logical that that might result in a bit of tenderness. Imagine stretching the little patch of skin between your thumb and forefinger every one to three hours constantly for three days. Or sucking on it with a bit of stretch. I think that might take a little bit of getting used to. There is some research that suggests discomfort for the first three to five days can be within normal range. UNICEF Baby friendly say you will experience a pulling sensation which 'may or may not' be painful. Pain is such a subjective thing so it's always going to be difficult to make hard and fast rules.

Do you feel a sharp pain that's deeper in your breast – behind the areola – about one to two minutes after breastfeeding has started? Does it feel a bit like an electrical tingle sometimes? This could be what we call 'let-down pains' and it's not connected to latching. When we get the milk ejection reflex, oxytocin arrives in the breast and contracts muscles around the milk storage areas to allow the milk to flow more quickly and push the milk down your ducts. This can be quite uncomfortable. Some women feel it strongly for the first few days or weeks and some women may never feel a letdown sensation. There's a big range of normal (we seem to say that a lot when it comes to breastfeeding!). Some people do a bit of googling and worry they might have thrush or an infection or something else is wrong but the letdown sensation can be a normal process and it only lasts for a few moments.

What wouldn't be normal is breastfeeding that results in a nipple coming out looking misshapen. It might come out looking longer but it shouldn't have a ridge across it, or be wedge-shaped or look like the end of an old lipstick. In the first few days, it might be uncomfortable as the nipple stretches but the rest of the feed should be manageable. You shouldn't be in the same level of pain throughout. The end of the feed shouldn't be worse than the beginning (that might mean the baby is slipping out of position and you need to look at your hold).

If your nipples start to become visibly cracked and

damaged; if you experience pain throughout a feed at the same level; if you are in pain after a feed; if your nipples are misshapen or white after a feed; if you start to dread the next feed – you need to get help. It isn't normal to be in pain after the first few days. If you've been pain-free for a while and suddenly things get harder, this could be the sign of an infection. We do sometimes find though, that after the first few weeks, mums can get sore again. This can be because they developed a way of holding their baby when they were teeny and now the baby is heavier, the weight of the baby is pulling down on mum's hands and arms and the baby is slipping. This may be imperceptible. It only has to be a pull of a few millimetres and things can start to get uncomfortable as the nipple is pressed against the hard palate or rubbed by the end of baby's tongue.

What helps sore nipples to heal? Sorting out the underlying problem. If you've been breastfeeding for a while and it becomes painful after a period of no difficulties at all, this might point to the possibility of an infection. This might be a bacterial infection like staph aureus or it could be a fungal infection. The nipple may look a bit pinker than usual, or shiny or be itchy or oozy

What helps sore nipples to heal?
Sorting out the underlying problem.

142

or have a yellow crust on it. Your doctor can take a swab and work out what's going on and you may be given a topical cream. If the nipple has a crack or is misshapen after a feed, perhaps there is an emerging latching issue. It's possible for things to change even if latching has been fine for ages. Babies get bigger and heavier and the shape of their mouth changes and they get teeth. There are a lot of variables. Just because your midwife says your latch 'was fine' (however long ago), that doesn't mean it might not be a problem now. In some cases, putting something on your nipples can help.

We used to say never to wash damaged nipples with soap and water. As the new edition of the La Leche League book, 'The Womanly Art of Breastfeeding' says, "Soap and Water is back!" We now know that soap and water is an important tool in fighting bacteria and preventing an infection like staph aureus. We need to break down any biofilm on the nipple (which is a grim word, let alone concept). There's a good overview here: http://www.cwgenna.com/nhygiene.html

If you have cracked or damaged nipples, we want to avoid a scab forming. We want to use a technique called 'moist wound healing'. Apply a thin layer of lanolin or Vaseline after a feed and this should enable you to heal from the inside out. Scabs get removed with each feed and leave nerve endings exposed. Once upon a time, mums were told to let damaged nipples dry out. Now we want to do the opposite. Some mums also apply breastmilk because it has antibacterial properties.

Complications: Feeling Low

This isn't specifically about breastfeeding or feeding but you may be reading this book and new motherhood feels like more of a struggle than it should.

We often have huge expectations of how motherhood is supposed to go. We know there are the jokes about not sleeping and being covered in baby milk but it seems a heck of a lot less funny when you've had less than twelve hours sleep in the last four days and you're scared to drive to the supermarket because it probably wouldn't be safe for you to get behind the wheel. This is meant to be magical and wonderful and you are filled with love and joy. Instead sometimes it feels scary and responsible and you might feel like you've lost yourself a little bit. EVERYONE has moments when they worry they aren't doing this right. It's also true that most people have periods of feeling tearful and overwhelmed. A few days after we've given birth, most women have a hormonal drop known as 'baby blues' when they may feel particularly low. It might be around the time you experience post-partum breast engorgement which is an unfortunately combination. Ideally this only lasts a few days but some people may need extra help.

Around 10% of new mums (and some new dads too) experience post-partum depression (also known as post-natal depression). If the feeling of being overwhelmed and low becomes too much, there are people who want to help you. We sometimes think depression is about feeling 'disconnected' and 'sad' but it can come in different forms. Some new mums may be too focused on baby's safety and terrified that something might go wrong. They might feel angry or lash out at others. If anything about your mood worries you, your health visitor or your GP can help. There are things that can be done. Some mums find talking therapy helpful and sometimes antidepressants which are compatible with breastfeeding can be given. Have a look at the PANDA website for more information. It can help enormously to find other mums online who understand what you are going through. Look for #PNDchat on Twitter.

We know that women who successfully breastfeed are less likely to experience depression but breastfeeding struggles or giving up breastfeeding after a period of difficulty might make things worse (http://www.cam. ac.uk/research/news/breastfeeding-linked-to-lower-risk-of-postnatal-depression). Another reason why it's really important to get help when breastfeeding doesn't seem to be going to plan.

A small group of breastfeeding mums experience something called D-MER. This is when the milk ejection reflex (when the milk lets down) does unhelpful things to dopamine and happy hormones in your brain and when you start to breastfeed, you actually experience a wave of anxiety/ sadness/ anger. It only lasts a few moments – minutes at worst – and doesn't even last throughout the entire feed. It's very rare but worth mentioning as it can knock you for six when it does happen. A lot of people take a while to get diagnosed and realise what is going on.

Complications: Flat or Inverted Nipples

If you have completely flat or inverted nipples will this make breastfeeding more difficult? The honest answer is 'probably not but you may need some extra help'. First of all, things can still change in pregnancy. Your breast shape and nipple shape change in response to pregnancy hormones and you may be surprised by how things end up looking. However, even if things don't change it's called 'breastfeeding' and not 'nipplefeeding' for a reason. A baby that is latched on well has a good mouthful of breast and uses their tongue to scoop the breast tissue towards the back of their mouth. You may need some extra help to get the positioning right so make an extra special effort to find local support. You may find it useful to shape your breast just prior to a feed perhaps by creating something called a 'nipple sandwich'. There are also some devices that help draw out the nipple and some make their own with a modified syringe. Some people wear breast shells before a feed to help draw out their nipple. Pumping for a few moments may also help. With a flat nipple, it may take a few more days to get used to the sensation of breastfeeding as your nipple will be stretched and shaped in baby's mouth. The most important thing is to understand that breastfeeding can work for you and women with flat and inverted nipples feed every day without any difficulty whatsoever.

Complications: Worried About Low Milk Supply

I'm guessing you are reading this because you are worried you may have low milk supply. I don't mean to doubt your situation but it's crucial to note that the MAJORITY of new mothers who fear they have low milk supply DO NOT. The majority of women who start to use formula because they worry they aren't making enough or baby isn't getting enough DO NOT HAVE A PROBLEM. I cannot emphasise this enough. Apologies for the capital letters.

Every day mothers panic and end breastfeeding or start using formula and there is not an underlying problem with their milk supply. But of course – once they start using formula without correct support, they often will start to send signals to their breasts to really reduce supply.

* You do not have low milk supply just because your baby won't go the X number of hours between feeds that the book on your coffee table tells you they should. Or your mother-in-law. Or the X number of hours your friend's baby is going between feeds. A normal happy healthy baby who has a gorgeous mummy with a normal healthy milk supply might get hungry an hour after the last feed, or ninety minutes, or forty-five minutes or two hours. They might be cluster feeding and hardly want to come off the breast

at all. They might be having a growth spurt and feed every hour for a day.

- You do not have low milk supply because your breasts have stopped leaking. Some mothers leak less than others. MOST mothers notice that leaking reduces at the weeks go by and the teeny tiny sphincter muscles responsible tighten.

- You do not have low milk supply because your breasts feel softer than they used to. The excessive fullness we experience in the early days of breastfeeding is about vascular engorgement (blood and lymph) and it's about the body inefficiently storing unnecessary amounts of milk between feeds. As time goes by, the breasts get cleverer at storage (don't forget milk is also made while a baby is actually feeding). There is also less blood and lymph needed in the breasts as breast tissue growth slows down. At the beginning, it's often very obvious which breast is going to be fed from next. That feeling goes. And many mothers mistakenly connect it with a reduction in milk supply. We are not all supposed to continue feeling heavy and full throughout our breastfeeding experience. Don't ever think "I'll wait to let my breasts fill up!" Noooooo. This shows a misunderstanding of how lactation works to a spectacular degree. When breasts are fuller, milk production slows down. When breasts are emptier, milk production increases. Emptier softer breasts may well be making a heap more milk in a 24 hour period than the engorged full versions.

- You do not have low milk supply because your baby feeds for a short time. Plenty of babies get everything they need in less than ten minutes. Probably not five – but sometimes a feed might even be five minutes long. Lots of babies use their tongue and jaw muscles super efficiently and gulp and glug and slow down as the milk gets fattier and thicker and then come off happy. It might take them nine minutes or nineteen. A baby might start off life needing thirty minutes to drain a breast (when we say 'drain', breasts are never completely empty, it just means the baby has taken out all the milk they usefully want to). As a baby gets older, this can dramatically reduce. It doesn't mean less milk is going in. If a small sleepy jaundiced baby falls asleep very quickly at the breast without some solid minutes of good swallowing, that's a different story. Overall however, a longer feed does not always mean a better one

- You do not have low milk supply because you have small breasts. Large breasts are a combination of fatty tissue and glandular tissue. You cannot tell much about someone's milk production by the size of the breasts. If you are really worried your breasts don't 'look right', we'll come back to this later.

- You do not have low milk supply just because your baby wakes up a lot. Plenty of young babies feed with similar intervals day and night. Plenty continue waking every two to three hours for a while.

- You do not have low milk supply because your baby

won't 'go down' after a feed. So you feed your baby and they drop off to sleep on the breast. You move them to the Moses basket and they wake up as if you just placed them on a sheet of molten lead. And they seem to be rooting again. This happens because being next to you skin-to-skin was nice and cosy and relaxing and warm and it smelt good. The Moses basket is cold and NOT YOU. You probably triggered the Moro startle reflex when you moved them. You probably moved them about fifteen to thirty minutes after a feed when the hormone cholecystokinin had dropped in their blood stream causing them to be more wakeful. Your teeny primate mammal baby finds the breast a lovely place to be. They like to suck to relax themselves. Babies like second helpings. This does not mean you are not making enough milk.

- You do not have low milk supply because your baby will take milk out of a bottle after a feed. Put a teat against a young baby's palate and you trigger that baby's sucking reflex. Babies will usually continue to take milk beyond the point that they need it. This is one of the reasons we see links between bottle-feeding and obesity.

- You do not have low milk supply because you don't pump very much milk. Pumping and breastfeeding are surprisingly unrelated. Your baby removes milk in a completely different way. Plenty of women with healthy milk supplies fail to pump much at all. Their bodies can't be tricked into eliciting the milk ejection reflex (or 'letdown'). Plus pumps don't always work. Suction goes as valves get old.

These are the things that REALLY tell you a mother might have low milk supply:

- Weight gain problems. A newborn is born and then loses weight. They regain birth weight at around two weeks. They then put on about 150-200g a week after that. That slows down after around four months. If your newborn loses more than 10% of their body weight, we might pay attention but we'll also want to look at things like your birth. Did you have a drip in labour that filled you and your baby with fluid? Did your gorgeous newborn look a wee bit like the Stay Puft marshmallow man in their first photos? That fluid elevated the birth weight and as it comes out again in the first few days, we might see more of a weight drop. That doesn't necessarily mean feeding or supply is a problem. However wouldn't want your baby to lose weight after about day five or lose weight a second time. It might take some babies three weeks to get back up to birth weight.

  Have a look at the chart in your red book. Notice how we have birth weight line and then a space where the curvy lines don't go and they start again at week two. Just because your baby was born on the 75th percentile, that doesn't mean we would expect them to definitely re-start on the 75th after that two week gap. That's why the lines don't continue. That's why we have that space. We start again at two weeks. Your baby might be on the 50th then. They then ideally will roughly stick in the same vicinity. But babies wobble around a bit. They might dip below. They might get close to the 25th. And then they might bob back up again. We don't expect all babies to hug a line exactly. This chart is a guide. It's about averages. It's not about mathematical certainties.

- Nappies. In the early days (first four weeks), we look at poo and pee. After your milk has come in (around day two to five), we'd expect to see six wet nappies in 24 hours and three poos the size of a £2 coin or bigger. After week four, some baby's poo rate can slow right down. This doesn't mean anything is wrong. Some babies can skip several days between poos and this isn't anything to do with milk transfer or supply. However if someone tells you it's OK for a ten day old baby not to poo for a few days, don't believe them. We'd need to investigate that situation. Only later on do we relax.

Weight gain and nappies. That's it. Those are the only things that tell us about milk supply. You may hear people say that 'babies should be settled after a feed' but some babies get wind or need to poo or have reflux or wake up and want second helpings. Let's be careful about even saying that. Let's look at weight gain and nappies.

So let's now assume you do have low milk supply. How many of you are still with me? I'm sorry if you are. I'm sorry if your baby only put on 60g last week and 90g or less or nothing the week before that and they are slipping down the percentiles. I'm sorry because I know how scary that can feel. Nothing feels like it matters more. There are things we can do.

1. Find people. Find people who know about breastfeeding. Someone who tells you just to use formula in this situation is not who you need. If that's all they can offer you, they don't know about breastfeeding and you need someone else. You need someone who understands how lactation works. These people may still tell you to use some formula in some situations (or donor breastmilk) but they will do so alongside telling you how to protect and develop your milk supply. You also need people close to you to look after you. If you are going to do all the other stuff on this list, you need to have people who love you who will cook your dinner and run you a bath sometimes. And text you just before the weigh-in clinic next week to say they are thinking of you.

2. Breastfeeding M.O.T. Someone like a breastfeeding counsellor or IBCLC (lactation consultant) should check your latch. You might not be sore and your nipples might not be misshapen after a feed but something still might be going wrong. Your latch needs checking. Is baby's chin deep into the breast?

Is baby's body close to yours? Is baby's ear/ shoulder/ hip in a line?

They shouldn't just check your latch but look at your breastfeeding management. Are you feeding enough? Maybe your baby doesn't show cues very strongly and someone told you to wait for them and you're sometimes going four hours between feeds? Maybe you need to feed more frequently?

When are you changing sides? Too quickly? (and baby is missing the fatty milk). OR did someone tell you to stick on one side forever to get that 'hind milk' and the baby is on forty-five minutes without doing a heck of a lot? Maybe you need to change sides at twenty to thirty minutes instead and get baby a greater volume of milk overall and fatty milk overall? Both of these habits can cause weight gain problems. Get someone to help you recognise what swallowing looks like so you'll know when to change sides and when good feeding has finished. Ask someone to check your baby for tongue tie.

3. Google 'breast compressions'. You'll get to a video and hand out from Dr Jack Newman. You can finish a feed with breast compressions and get an extra dose of fatty milk into baby.

4. You have three sides and four sides. This is 'switch nursing'. Try and go back to the first side. There will be milk there. The more breastfeeding you do, the more milk you will make. The second time you return to that breast, the milk will be fattier and richer and

you'll send great signals to your body to make more.

5. Find time. If you are going to build up your supply, get help. You can't devote time to switch nursing and skin-to-skin when you have to go to Tesco to buy milk and pick up another child from school. If this is 'Operation Milk supply', who can help you? You'll read people talking about a 'babymoon'. Go to bed, they say. Just you and the baby. Feed lots. If that sounds appealing, go for it. Personally my babymoon would involve the sofa and box sets and crisps. However there's no point in babymoooning until next Christmas if your latch and breastfeeding management are the issues. Get that checked first.

6. Using a pump. Baby feeding effectively is first choice but pumps can be useful. You can pump on an emptier breast to send even more signals to your milk supply. But we're not going to take a baby off the breast do be able to pump.

   You don't need to wash and sterilize a pump every time you use it. Pop it in a plastic bag and put it back into the fridge between pumping sessions. Wash and sterilize once in 24 hours. Ten minutes for each pumping session is ample. If you are pumping for thirty minutes and 'nothing is coming' out, you are not getting a letdown and you are not doing yourself any favours. Use hand expression before and after (google 'Marmet hand expression') and prepare the breasts with warm compresses and massage if you can. You can take an hour and do some 'cluster pumping' or 'power pumping'. Pretend to be a baby having a cluster feed. Pump for ten minutes. Break for five. Pump again and repeat.

Just check your pump is the best one available. If it's second hand or you have had it a while, it might need servicing or replacement parts. You also might want to consider hiring a hospital grade double electric pump from someone like www.ardobreastpumps. co.uk to give yourself the opportunity to pump both sides together as effectively as possible.

Pumping shouldn't hurt. Make sure your flanges are the right size – that means they are the right diameter for the size of your nipple. Don't think that cranking up the suction will automatically do better things. And don't think, "I don't want to pump because I will empty my breasts and baby will have less milk." Certainly they might be less appreciative if you pump just before a feed is due and you leave them with an emptier breast full of thicker fattier milk but pumping overall will increase milk supply and stimulate milk production. You are not 'taking their milk away'.

You might also be someone who always gets better results with just using hand expression so stick with that. Of course, you might not want to pump at all and just focus on feeding baby more effectively and frequently.

7. Galactagogues. Taking herbs and medication that increase milk supply. Not right for everyone but some women really feel they helped. You need to read

about side effects and dosage on sites like kellymom. com. Fenugreek, blessed thistle and goat's rue are popular. Some doctors prescribe domperidone or metoclopramide in certain situations. These are never a substitute for good breast emptying and a breastfeeding MOT.

8. The science part. In a book, this bit would be under a little flap as we're only talking to a small group of people.

Did you have breast surgery?

Are your breasts very widely-spaced or asymmetrical, or very tubular with a bulging areola? Did they not really change much in pregnancy (or puberty)?

Do you have PCOS? Some women with PCOS (not all) have a reduced milk supply.

These are times when it's worth finding an IBCLC and getting technical.

Some doctors will do hormonal testing for you. There are medications that can help develop breast tissue especially in pregnancy.

What about your thyroid levels? This is something relevant for more people than you might realise. If you are trying everything and low milk supply continues to be a problem, ask your doctor to check your thyroid levels. There are sometimes medical reasons mothers have a low milk supply and doctors and lactation consultants may be able to help you. These are not the most common reasons why people have low milk supply by a long shot. Hence the need for the flap.

Most people who genuinely have low milk supply got themselves into a pickle with using artificial nipples or not breastfeeding enough or breastfeeding ineffectively. And it can almost always be reversed.

Also remember that just because you had low milk supply in your first breastfeeding experience, it doesn't mean a subsequent lactation will also be a struggle. The development of all that breast tissue first time round often helps.

Hold in your mind the fact that women can relactate after not breastfeeding at all for several weeks. We CAN send signals to increase supply again in the vast majority of cases. There are tons of us in real life and online who want to support you.

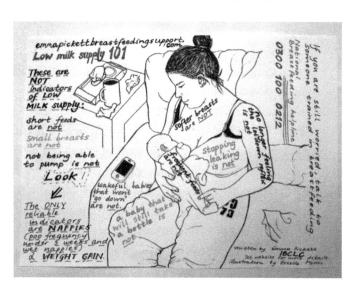

A Message for Partners

I am constantly struck by the vital role the non-breastfeeding partner plays in this story. I hope your partner is reading the books too. I hope they are attending the breastfeeding class and listening to descriptions of positioning and attachment. I hope they get why this is important and why they are important.

I wrote the article below one afternoon after coming back from a consult.

The Breastfeeding Dad
(and this also applies to breastfeeding partners who are not 'dads' but a second mum).

I worked with a new family for the second time today. I won't go into too much detail but things aren't going well with breastfeeding and mum is in a lot of discomfort.

As I left them today with plans to see them next week, I knew absolutely that the dad was holding them all together. I am not doubting the determination or commitment of that brand new mother recovering from her difficult birth and finding life was tough, but that father – of only a few days – had precisely the strength that his new family needed.

He sat quietly while she described her experiences and her perception of what was going wrong. He gently prompted and corrected when it was appropriate to do so and all the time he gave off this force that said, "I know we can do this. I know this is the best thing. We are going to make this work." He actually said out loud, "We believe in this."

At one point the mum was concerned she might not be able to go on and he said softly, "The low point was two nights ago. You've come really far since then. Things are getting better," and he explained how. And she said, "Yeah, you're right," and calmed immediately.

He praised her without being sappy. He took the baby to calm him at just the right moments. He listened carefully to what was discussed because he knew he was part of this breastfeeding thing too.

He knew that in the middle of the night, when she felt she just couldn't cope, it mattered that he'd paid attention to the right positioning and latching. Not least because sometimes it really helps to have that second pair of eyes looking from a different angle and observing whole body position.

Let's just assume for practical purposes that this bloke must be a prat in other ways as no one could be that perfect – however he absolutely knew how to be a breastfeeding dad.

And I see a lot of dads like that.

It's surprisingly often that it's dad who calls the National Breastfeeding Helpline. It's clear something wasn't going right and for whatever reason mum couldn't face making that call. So dad does and almost always manages to get mum on the phone in the end.

And it's dads who research where the breastfeeding

groups are, phone the lactation consultants, get the troops lined up when things aren't going well. They give mum the space she needs and over and over again manage to manoeuvre the support just when it's needed. Yes, sure, some of that is because men like to try and solve problems. They see a difficulty and want to fix it in the face of feeling somewhat helpless. But these same 'helpless men' come to consultations and express their worries while empowering and supporting their wives at the same time. It's a subtle and impressive skill. Especially when you're sleep-deprived.

Dads use some of that diplomacy even when things are going well with breastfeeding. Most new parents today weren't breastfed themselves as infants in the 1970s and 1980s. We are the generation of the formula-feeding grannies. Some of those older women become awesome champions of breastfeeding and some struggle to witness something they don't understand. The dads are the knights at the gatehouse – letting through only the right support. They act as the barrier between new mum and mother-in-law who might not know when to step back. They make sure that the new mum and baby can make the nest they need to.

Breastfeeding dads might be good at nappies and burping and baths and making sandwiches and passing the remote control but that's a tiny slice of what they can do. They can provide a bedrock where a new mother learns how she wants to be a new mother and where breastfeeding can flourish.

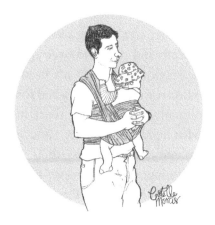

What About a Lesbian Partner?

You may be supporting your partner – the birth mother – to breastfeed while you carve out your own way to be a new mummy. Your role in supporting your partner to breastfeed is essential. Perhaps you might consider breastfeeding too. You may be 'inducing lactation' for yourself. Even if you haven't been pregnant and have never been pregnant, it is possible for you to develop a milk supply and breastfeed. If you want to read more about it, you can do so here.

http://www.prideangel.com/p183/fertility-pregnancy/Induced-Lactation.aspx

This is an article I wrote for the website Pride Angel. I've also advised couples in person who are interested in induced lactation and you should find the same support from many lactation consultant and breastfeeding counsellors. You need to get started several months before baby arrives though if you are going to follow the process fully and give yourself the best chance to build a milk supply.

Breastfeeding and Your Relationship

I should just warn you that what follows will include some discussion of SEX.

I'm sometimes asked, "Why don't more people in the UK breastfeed until six months?" Obviously the reasons are complex. It's often about people not being able to access the breastfeeding support they need in the first month. It's also often about new parents not realising what's normal when it comes to breastfeeding and being surrounded by a bottle-feeding culture that undermines their confidence. However I think a little bit of it is connected to the way British women think about their breasts and their bodies. I think a little bit of it might be because we don't know how to be a breastfeeding mum and be a sexual partner at the same time.

From when we are very small, we are surrounded by the message that boobs are about sex. We see it on billboards, in daily newspapers, on magazine covers. Think of all the images an average twenty year old woman will have received about her breasts and how many of those images are about a woman feeding her baby. And that's just the girls – never mind the new fathers.

We are bombarded with all these messages about what breasts are 'for' and then we're told when we're pregnant, "Oh, by the way, forget all that, THIS is REALLY what breasts are for. It's really important. It's best for baby. OK?" It's quite a brain shift.

We live in a society where we no longer live in extended families and the couple is the centre of our household. Successful couples in our culture are couples with active sex lives and sometimes when we are a new parent, we're finding our way when it comes to sex. We're trying to work out how to be a mother and how to be a sexual partner at the same time. Meanwhile dad (or partner) is trying to figure out how to support you in your new role as a mother and understands this teeny new person is your new priority. But they would quite like to feel loved as well. I never subscribe to the view that breastfeeding makes new dads feel excluded. But when there's a new baby at the centre of your world and dad is shunted back to work after only two weeks of paternity leave while you carry on getting to know this new person, it's tough.

Sex isn't just about sex. It's a way for people to feel connected and loved and special. When you partner is asking for sex, it's not just about wanting to get his 'rocks off'. Most adult males (and females) are pretty proficient at organising the offing of rocks all by themselves. It's also about want to connect with you and feel that he still matters and your relationship as a couple still matters.

It's very easy when you are a new mum to get into a downward spiral of feeling negatively about sex and sex starting to feel like another chore. New motherhood is a time when you may actually find yourself using the cheesy expression 'touched out'. A little person is touching and needing us all day long. New motherhood is exhausting. If we feel 'needed' by anyone else who might place physical demands on us, it can feel like a step too far.

Not to mention the fact that after the birth we may have physical reasons for not feeling quite ready for sex. There is some suggestion that breastfeeding can result in lower oestrogen levels and this might result in increased levels of vaginal dryness. This may be true for some women in the early months and lubrication can be useful. Although some may claim that breastfeeding 'affects your hormones' in a way that impacts on libido, it's difficult to make any hard and fast rules when it comes to libido. In pregnancy, we all have fairly similar hormones flying around and some women feel very sexual and motivated and others switch off sex entirely. Whatever might be causing sex to feel difficult for some new mothers, we need to be conscious of what's going on and recognise that we need to spare a bit of mental energy for our relationship.

When it comes to protecting and cherishing your relationship there are some things that are worth spelling out:

- Everyone is more tired and we aren't always brilliant communicators when we are tired. We may be snappier and less patient and need to be more conscious of the words we are choosing and the way we are saying things.

- It's worth pausing and taking a moment to think through what's really important. If your partner doesn't put on a baby's nappy in exactly the same way you might, that might be a comment worth letting go. In the beginning, you were both muddling through this parenting thing together but as the hours went by you probably spent more and more time with the baby and they possibly felt more excluded and disempowered. You simply had more practice. It is your job to mother your child but also to empower your partner to be a new parent in the best way you can. OK, if they are rrrreally bad at putting the nappy on, you can say something.

- There may be new ways to be intimate. In the olden days (a few weeks ago before baby), it might have seemed logical for couple time to consist of evenings out, dinner in a restaurant and sex before falling asleep in bed. These are often spectacularly bad ways for a couple to try and reconnect when they have a new teeny baby. Evenings and bedtimes are the times when we may feel the most exhausted. There are also often the times when baby wants to cluster feed and is at their most demanding. Whereas 9pm once felt like the beginning of an exciting evening, it now feels like a time when your body is pretty convinced it really shouldn't have to be operating fully conscious. We may have to rethink what 'couple time' means. Time as a couple doesn't have to mean time separated from baby. It is possible for the three of you to curl up on the sofa and watch a great movie, or go for a walk in a beautiful place, or have a nice meal in a restaurant. Young babies sleep and when they don't sleep, they breastfeed and that tends to be peaceful and straightforward. You might prefer to be in that restaurant at 6pm or 2pm instead of 9pm. If you are ready for time away from baby (and don't force yourself until it feels right – this isn't a test of anything), take care with who you choose to look after your baby. It may be that your first meal out isn't with your partner at all because that's who you first trust to be at home with baby while you eat out with a friend. When it comes time for the babysitter to give you couple time, it might make sense for the babysitter to be there from 2pm to 7pm giving you a chance for a meal and an experience and still get home for bed. Or how about a babysitter who takes the baby to park or a family member who takes baby to their own home while you and your partner share a bath and have some intimate time? Or how about you share a bath and have some intimate time with a baby in a Moses basket nearby? You can be both things at once – a mother and a partner. We feel we have to compartmentalise ourselves and that just isn't true.

No one has to 'switch off' being a mother in order to be intimate and connect with their partner. And intimate time doesn't have to mean putting a penis into a vagina. There are lots of options that you can talk about honestly. If communication is open, you don't have to avoid other physical affection because you fear that you are sending signals you are ready for sex when you aren't.

- Talk. Sometimes we feel that new parenthood is supposed to be lovely and we're supposed to be thrilled and grateful and jolly. The reality is that it's very difficult. Any relationship with weak points is likely to find those weak points even more exposed. It's a time to communicate honestly and kindly.

- You do have to make time for your partner. Don't roll your eyes at me for spelling that out. (You may think "I hardly have time to brush my teeth so get stuffed.") Truthfully, your baby benefits from parents who are connected and loving. Do you find yourself feeling angry towards your partner more than you feel loving and appreciative? You may need to talk more. Taking time to listen to your partner and show kindness is for all of you as a family. A bestselling baby writer suggests women drink a large glass of red wine and force themselves to have sex even when they don't feel like it. If this is what sex has come to mean to you, you need to talk more with your partner and use a bit more imagination. One of the symptoms of postnatal depression is a feeling of resentment towards your partner, a disinterest in sex and a lack of motivation in reconnecting. It might be that your partner is simply a complete prat and all these feelings are justified. Some relationships may breakdown in the first few months after a baby is born and that might not be a bad thing. However if you feel that life isn't quite going the way you'd like in other ways too, take a moment to talk to someone about how you feel and just check you don't need further help.

- Be kind to yourself. Our bodies change when we are new mums. They are supposed to. That can feel weird when we are surrounded by magazines and images telling us that flat tummies are the meaning of life and breasts aren't about babies. Breastfeeding itself doesn't make your breasts sag, by the way. That is the effect of pregnancy hormones and may happen to people who don't breastfeed even for a minute. Breastfeeding may make inverted nipples evert for ever more but it's not going to permanently change your breasts. And even if it did make a little alteration, most women would feel it was more than

Be kind to yourself too. Our bodies change when we are new mums. They are supposed to.

worth it for the all the positives – including reducing a mother's risk of breast cancer. If you feel you want to lose weight, that can still happen while you are breastfeeding. Have a look at 'diet' in the section 'Can I do this if I'm breastfeeding?' Breastfeeding mums can still run and play netball and swim in the sea. Just don't push yourself to do too much too fast because you feel you need to rush to change your body back into the way it was. Your baby will only be a baby for a short time. Before you know it, it will be all about finding shoes and reading stories and playing football and banging drums and wearing sparkly dresses. Your priority right now is meeting this new person and getting to know them and caring for them and taking on probably the most important role of your life.

For a discussion on contraception and breastfeeding, have a look at 'Can I do this if I'm breastfeeding?'

A Message for Grandparents

You might not know that it's normal for a breastfed baby to want to feed even though they only fed an hour ago. Or that a breastfed baby might cluster feed in the evenings and feed continually for a block of time even though breastfeeding is going well and mum's supply is great. You might not realise that the best way you can help is not by offering to feed the baby but by taking the baby after a feed so mum can nap and promising to wake her if baby needs to feed again. What we know about breastfeeding has been transformed over the last few decades. When ultrasound started to become a useful tool, we could look inside live lactating breasts for the first time. We learnt about issues like the variety in storage capacity and that some women may never be able to leave it three hours between feeds and if they did try, they could damage their milk supply and cause lasting problems.

If you are a grandparent, your job is to mother the parent and not the baby. Your role is to empower the new parent and allow them to come to trust their own instincts. You empower them by allowing them to find their own solutions and supporting their decisions.

By all means call the helplines, read the books and ask the questions. If you are informed, you may well be able to provide useful support. Your best bet is to help the new parents to reach the information themselves.

We know that introducing a bottle too early can jeopardise a baby's ability to latch onto the breast effectively. Early bottle use is connected to earlier cessation of breastfeeding. Pumping and bottle-feeding can also adjust a mum's milk supply at a time when baby should be sending the necessary signals. The best way to support practically is to hold a sleeping baby who doesn't want to put down between feeds, burp and nappy change before doing any feeding. You can feed the parents.

A new parent needs to trust that you understand their

*If you are a grandparent, your job
is to mother the parent and not the
baby. Your role is to empower the new
parent and allow them to come to trust
their own instincts*

role as the decision-maker. It will be frustrating at times as the guidance given today will differ greatly from what was said twenty or even ten years ago. Research is producing a new evidence-base for clinical and healthcare advice all the time.

There may be times when you come to reflect on your own parenting choices and wonder whether you could have done things differently. It's only recently that we've come to understand much more about how breastfeeding and milk production works. Many women in the 1970s, 80s and 90s had their own breastfeeding experience sabotaged by incorrect information and misleading advice. This can be difficult to deal with when it may only sink in when you see your child parenting differently. You may be subconsciously affected by the decisions you made and seeing your grandchild being parented differently. If you feel frustrated or confused, step away and take some time to reflect. The helplines are really happy to have calls from new grandparents and you can ask questions about any aspect of breastfeeding.

You will be a crucial person in this breastfeeding journey. Your encouragement and practical help with be incredibly important. Thank you for reading this and showing that you already understand the part you will be playing. It will be appreciated by new parents and all of us who try to support them. We know how much grandparents matter in helping to make breastfeeding work.

Can I Do This If I'm Breastfeeding?

Can I eat soft cheese, sushi, cold meats? YES! Almost everything you couldn't eat in pregnancy is now fine. There may still be a small risk of contamination or food poisoning but baby is not at risk in the same way and if you get ill, your breastmilk will provide protection for baby.

Can I eat swordfish, marlin, oily fish? Yes, but you need to eat it in moderation. Not everyone knows this but two portions of week of oily fish and no more than one portion of shark, swordfish or marlin. (Please tell me you're not actually eating shark). This is because of the build-up of pollutants and heavy metals including dioxins and PCBs. In pregnancy, you were told to limit tuna. This is not considered necessary when breastfeeding: (http://www.nhs.uk/chq/Pages/should-pregnant-and-breastfeeding-women-avoid-some-types-of-fish.aspx?CategoryID=54). You'll be relieved to hear gurnard and flounder are among the fish not to worry about.

Can I get my nails painted and dye my hair? Yes! (http://www.breastfeedingnetwork.org.uk/wp-content/dibm/beauty-treatments-oct-14.pdf)

You can even get a fake tan though I'm honestly not sure that would taste great and I have seen an amusing photo on the internet of a toddler with fake tanned cheeks so exercise caution.

Can I get a tattoo? Most tattoo artist professionals will not knowingly tattoo a woman who is pregnant or who is breastfeeding. There is a risk of infection and reaction. It is certainly crucial that you use a proper tattoo artist who is licenced and practising proper infection control. Hepatitis, HIV and tetanus could all be spread if universal precautions are not being used. (http://www.llli.org/faq/tattoos.html)

Can I drink alcohol? Yes, some. A younger and smaller baby is more likely to be affected. It is not advisable to drink to excess (especially if you are caring for a baby) and it's not a good idea to drink any alcohol and then share your bed with a baby. However having some alcoholic drinks occasionally is not a reason to stop breastfeeding nor to end exclusive breastfeeding. One to two units once or twice a week is probably OK. It takes around two hours for a unit of alcohol to leave your blood stream. It's going to peak about thirty minutes after a drink depending on how much you've eaten and your body mass. The levels in your milk match what's in your blood and you don't need to pump out the milk with the alcohol in it. It will naturally reduce as it levels your bloodstream. People don't realise that milk is constantly made and reabsorbed. You may want to pump though if you are getting engorged or to protect your supply if you are not feeding for a short time. You could give a bottle of milk you have expressed earlier if you are concerned you shouldn't be feeding. I've heard someone say the best time to drink is while you are actually feeding as the alcohol won't have entered your bloodstream and it will be the maximum interval before you need to feed again!

Can I take this medication? The answer is usually yes. There are very few medications which are not compatible with breastfeeding. It's sad to say that many doctors and nurses struggle to get access to up-to-date evidence-based information when it comes to medication and breastfeeding. There are still mothers being told they need to 'pump and dump' after a general anaesthetic when mums who've had a C-section will breastfeed a much smaller baby immediately on waking up. Many drug companies will say that a drug isn't automatically safe during breastfeeding because to say otherwise gives them a legal responsibility for your safety. It's much easier to say that you need to speak to a doctor. A good place to find out more information is the Breastfeeding Network site. They have a selection of useful factsheets: (http://www.breastfeedingnetwork.org.uk/detailed-information/drugs-in-breastmilk/). Another excellent resource is the 'Drugs in Breastmilk' service run by the Breastfeeding Network. You can message them through their Facebook page or email them. This service has saved many breastfeeding relationships in the face of poor information. You can also buy apps for your smart phone like 'LactMed' and 'Infant Risk Center' (which contains information from Dr Thomas Hale who is one of the world's leading experts on breastmilk and medication).

Can I eat junk food? If you eat burgers for breakfast, lunch and tea with crisps for dessert and cream cakes for starters, breastfeeding is still the best choice for your baby a thousand times over. Our lactation is surprisingly robust. Your supply won't disappear if you don't eat well for a few days. The 'quality' of your milk won't be affected because you skipped a few meals and don't like vegetables. The fat we lay down in pregnancy is there as a store for the milk we produce and research shows that women living in communities with access to poorer diets will still produce good quality milk. We may suffer first if we eat poorly or not enough. Our bodies will prioritise lactation.

The best plan is to eat when you are hungry and drink when you are thirsty. There is some evidence that forcing yourself to drink lots of water can actually reduce your supply slightly rather than increasing it. You just need to drink enough to keep your urine pale. If you eat natural and healthy foods, you may feel better for it but you don't need to eat large amounts in addition to what you might eat otherwise. The charity 'First Steps Nutrition' produced a guide you may find useful: http://www.firststepsnutrition.org/newpages/Infants/infant_feeding_eating_well_breastfeeding_mothers.html

Can I drink coffee? Yes, you can. Some babies are affected by caffeine more than others so you may have to experiment and see what happens. Research seems to suggest that the upper limit is somewhere around 300mg a day. A cup of tea contains about 48mg and one cup of filter coffee is about 100mg. A can of coke has about 45mg.

Can I still lose weight and diet? Yes, you can. Though you need to make sure you still have enough energy – not just for making milk but also for the business of being a new parent. You need a mixed diet and ideally not lose more than 1-2 pounds a week and try not to drop your calorie intake too suddenly. You'll still need to expect to eat at least 1500-1800 calories each day. Dipping below that may impact on your supply. It also seems sensible to wait at least 6-8 weeks before starting a diet. You need to recover from birth and give your milk supply a chance to get established. It's also not a time to look for quick fixes like liquid diets.

Can I get pregnant if I'm breastfeeding? Sometimes. It's going to depend how old your baby is and how often you are breastfeeding. Nature isn't daft. Human babies are vulnerable and if a mum is feeding a young baby regularly, it wouldn't be sensible in terms of the survival of the species for us to regain fertility immediately. Doing *any* breastfeeding isn't enough to stop someone getting pregnant though. Ovulation can return while we are breastfeeding and we can develop the conditions for a fertilised egg to implant and do its thing. However if a baby is LESS than six months old; if your periods have not returned and if you are exclusively breastfeeding (no bottles, dummies, food), there is a good chance that this will be 98% effective as a method of contraception. It's called 'LAM' (Lactational Amenorrhoea Method). Amenorrhoea means you aren't having periods.

You need to be breastfeeding during the day and night and probably not going longer than about five hours between feeds at night and four hours in the day.

If this doesn't apply to you, you'll need to choose another method of contraception. You can read about some options here:

http://breastfeedingnetwork.org.uk/wp-content/dibm/contraception%20for%20website%20%283%29.pdf

Some women find their milk supply is affected by hormonal contraception so take some time to do some reading and find a method that makes you feel comfortable.

It is possible (though a lot less likely) to get pregnant before your period has returned. Some people talk about 'catching the first egg'. This sometimes happens when women are feeding older babies and toddlers.

It's also possible to be having a period and to not yet be fully fertile so if you are breastfeeding and want to get pregnant again, learn about the signs of ovulation and you may want to talk about someone about things you can do – like extending your luteal phase (the gap between your egg being released and your period where a fertilised egg has a chance to get properly stuck in).

By the way, you can conceive and go through your

entire pregnancy while still breastfeeding. We call it 'tandem feeding'. The only women not recommended to do this are those also advised to not have sex because their pregnancy is high risk. Extra oxytocin from breastfeeding may have a similar effect for these women. Your body 'resets' your milk supply back to colostrum so it can mean your older nursling has some runny poos but for many people that's the only downside. Once the new baby is born it can be a special thing to be feeding both of them and a way for baby and toddler to be connected. It doesn't feel right for everyone but I've yet to meet someone who did it who regretted it.

Twins and Multiples

As the title of this book and introduction convey, I believe a lot of breastfeeding success is down to self-belief and a determination to make it happen. We live in a society which undermines our efforts and we have to stand up to those voices that emphasise timings between feeds and how a baby should be sleeping and how long they should be feeding and how you should be running a 5K on Saturday morning after fixing your partner a frittata (not a euphemism).

This is even more true when we talk about mums of multiples. Those who have only had singletons watch from the periphery while mums pregnant with twins are told, "Rather you than me!", "Wow! I hope you've got support!", "How long while Bob have off work?", "Are you going to get a nanny/ maternity nurse?"

And if you are brave enough to mention you might be breastfeeding, "Don't try and do too much! Be realistic! Look after yourself! My hairdresser's sister's vicar's neighbour had twins and tried to breastfeed and she couldn't make it work!"

As if rolling over and unclipping a breastfeeding bra is soooo much harder than getting out of bed, boiling water, allowing it to cool for 70c while you find a sterilised bottle, mixing, cooling further and all the additional winding. Then you have to get babies back to sleep without the benefit of sleepy hormones like oxytocin and then get back to sleep yourself without those hormones that affect you too.

On what planet does anyone think that is easier?

Hey, mum of twins, I can get you two milk factories

You know that golden retriever lying snoozing while her ten puppies wriggle around and settle themselves into feeding? She's all blissed out with hormones? That could be you but with chocolate and Game of Thrones.

that you wear on your chest and they make milk constantly and it's always the right temperature and it contains about a gabillion medical benefits that I could spend hours telling you about. And you get to sit and lie with your babies and it helps your uterus contract and it helps you get back in shape. And your babies are less likely to suffer from reflux and digestive issues. And it doesn't cost money to put those factories there because they just get made automatically. In fact turning them off is more of a pain, and it hurts to do so.

Who would turn down that offer? Who is not at least going to try?

You know that golden retriever lying snoozing while her ten puppies wriggle around and settle themselves into feeding? She's all blissed out with hormones? That could be you but with chocolate and Game of Thrones.

And look at that golden retriever. Look at all those rows of nipples! Her body was clearly expecting a lot of babies. Her mammary glands don't look THAT big when you compare them to her body size and think of all the babies she is feeding! Where's all the milk? It looks like she must making milk as she goes along. Her breasts aren't just containers for storage. And sometimes she bats her babies away when she needs to get a drink of water or pee but basically her babies just feed when they need to while she relaxes too.

If you are going to get some help, it's a good idea to get people to feed *you* and look after your home. Have people who empower you to develop your relationship with your babies and know that breastfeeding twins is normal and ordinary.

Puppies' mum has ten teats. Human mummies have two. Why would we imagine that feeding two wasn't possible and we weren't going to make enough milk? Breastmilk production operates on a supply and demand basis. If two babies are demanding (in a loving and cute way) then mum's body will be supplying in the *majority of cases*. You'll know things are going OK because you'll be keeping an eye on nappies and weight gain.

At the beginning, things might be tougher as you're more likely to give birth to premature or smaller babies so you may need to get pumping. Your babies may even stay in hospital for a short while or be tube fed (with a nasal gastric tube). None of this is a barrier to successfully breastfeeding. Find people who know about breastfeeding and get pumping.

With premature babies, it is even more important that they receive breastmilk as there are some serious conditions that are more prevalent among premature babies who don't.

It's a good idea to talk to some people while you are pregnant. The breastfeeding organisations should be able to put you in touch with mums who have breastfed twins successfully. The ABM has breastfeeding counsellors who have fed twins for example. TAMBA is also a good resource and they have trained peer supporters. More from TAMBA here: https://www.tamba.org.uk/Parenting/First-Year/Feeding

It's good to talk through things like, "When it is better to feed a twin alone or should I always try and feed together?" That's going to depend on latching skills (theirs and yours). Sometimes it's initially easier to practice feeding just one but the other can have skin-to-skin meanwhile. You may find that very quickly you can feed them both at the same time though babies are likely to have different needs and wants and not being able to do feeds together is not a failure in any way. All families work out things a little differently. Two spare adults immediately post-birth are sensible. You need someone to look after you too.

In pregnancy, ask mums of twins online or in real life, "What positions work well?", "Would a special pillow be a good idea?", "What do you wish you'd known before the babies arrived?"

Mums can feed more than twins too. I came across a mum online two days ago who happily and successfully fed her triplets until they were two. Two days before that someone told me of a mum who breastfed quads (though her mother and sister did move in with her to help!)

If you can afford it (and even if you can't, don't assume this isn't an option available to you because there are ways round it), a doula can be a very precious thing to a new family with twins. Doulas offer your practical and emotional support during birth and the period afterwards. Crucially they do so while empowering you to become a new parent and skilling you rather than de-skilling you. You can read more here: http://doula.org.uk/

Positioning and Attachment Recap

You'll hear two different messages about positioning and attachment (how you hold the baby and how you latch them on to the breast) that seem to contradict each other. On the one hand, baby is filled with natural reflexes and you are too and you are both created for this breastfeeding business. When baby comes out, they just instinctively know what to do, if you can just tap into those instincts. If you simply lie back, a newborn baby will wiggle themselves into position (see videos of the breast crawl on YouTube).

Yet there's another message coming through. Breastfeeding seems like an exact science. Mothers have to think about angles of mouth and hard palates and soft palates and size of gapes and catching gapes at the right moment and holding baby in a particular way. It's like learning to drive except the gear stick is wriggly and cries a lot. It's left brain and right brain, not just a case of letting Mother Nature and her cosmic power flow over you.

These two messages seem completely at odds with each other. What's true?

Well, like most things, it's all a bit true. Some babies and mums do just seem to 'get it'. It's never sore. It's easy. It works.

However some mums need to take a bit more control over positioning. Perhaps some of baby's instincts haven't quite come to the surface because birth was a bit complicated. Perhaps first breastfeeding experiences didn't go well and it took a few days to get up and running. Perhaps you don't start out quite right (maybe that breastfeeding pillow wasn't such a great idea?) and now you need to concentrate a bit more to make things comfortable. Perhaps you just need to take charge a bit more and it's not quite clear why. You may not be able to predict beforehand exactly how your breastfeeding experience is going to go. You may have to wait and see what happens.

Whether you are in the nature-led or 'mother-led' group when it comes to positioning and attachment, there are certain positions that seem to be used by most people. It's a good idea to get pictures in your head now and even embarrass your partner by practising with a doll. Although be warned a doll doesn't have that flexible neck and that heavy head and that gorgeous biscuit baby smell. Your bump is also going to make things different.

The most important thing to remember is that one position isn't automatically better than all the others. Although it is a good idea to start off by giving recline/laid-back breastfeeding a go before moving on to more upright positions. You might work with a breastfeeding supporter who has a favourite and encourages you to try one position and then the next person to walk in the door could have another suggestion. As long as the key features are there, there are lots of options. You need that big wide mouth, the tongue extending and chin touching the breast. Their bottom lip will be flanged down (though you don't want to fiddle around too much to check or you'll mess things up). Their cheeks will be touching the breast and you may not be able to see their lips at all. You need baby's body nice and close to yours without their neck or body being twisted. Remember the ear/ shoulder/ hip all in a line. You need to be comfortable: your hands, arms and back.

Reclined position

When you lie back, with the baby on their tummy on top of you, it often seems to tap into some of their natural instincts and perhaps some of yours too. Sometimes when a baby has been really struggling to latch or even refusing entirely, lying right back and using the 'biological nurturing' position can make all the difference. We can give our arms a rest. We don't have to worry about how to hold their head, whether we're holding it too firmly, how that might feel for them after a difficult birth. Have a look at www.biologicalnurturing.com. Babies will often self-attach and mum might just raise an arm to keep a baby in place and prevent them toppling off if they sway. Just respond to baby's movements and help them wiggle into place if they are struggling. If you've had a C-section it might be more uncomfortable if baby's feet are placing against your scar so you may need to think more carefully about where the legs go but it's a great position because you don't have to sit up straight. First you'll need to lift baby onto your body (or get someone else to) and place their nose roughly around the nipple area and see what happens. Have their arms placed up either side of their upper body to help them stabilise themselves rather than down by their hips. It might look as if they are in a nearly crawling position. They may bob around and lift their

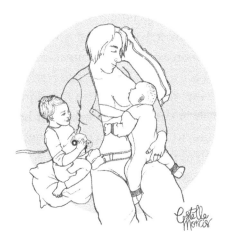

head up and then plonk it back down again. You may not be able to see very much in terms of latching. It might a feel like you are a bit out of control. It can still be a great position and sometimes it's worth lying back (literally) and seeing what your baby can do on their own. Wait a while to give baby time to work things out for themselves. Be patient. If it feels right to lend them a helping hand, do so and see what happens. In this position on their tummy, baby feels anchored and secure. Their arms don't flail around. They can get on with their job. Read Nancy Mohrbacher's article on this position: http://www. mothering.com/articles/natural-breastfeeding.

Rugby-Hold
The rugby hold or football hold (when North Americans are writing about it) can be a good choice particularly

when babies are little. Depending on your body shape and the shape of your breast, baby may be lying on their back or on their side or on a diagonal at your side. Importantly, baby shouldn't have to twist their neck to reach the breast. Remember the ear/ shoulder/ hip in a line thing? If your breasts are larger, it's more likely baby will be on their back. Remember to start with nose-to-nipple. If you start with mouth to nipple, the baby won't do that lovely head tilt that brings the chin to the breast. The important thing with this position is that you want the head tilt so that the chin isn't tucking into baby's chest. The baby's head should be stretched away from their chest. You try and drink a glass of water and swallow with your head tilted down! You'll be supporting baby's head by holding them roughly around their ears. Part of your hand will be around the top of their back. You're supporting their neck and the base of their head but you're not putting pressure

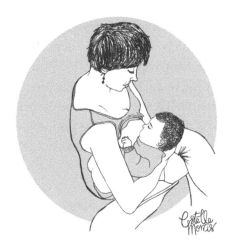

on their head. It's a supportive but gentle hold. If they want to tip back, they can. If you put pressure anywhere, it'll be on the top of their back to keep their chin tucked in close to the breast. Your arm should be supported probably by a cushion. It's not easy to do this position with baby dangling in mid-air. This position is often good if baby has a tongue restriction or if baby hasn't been doing really wide gapes in a cradle or cross-cradle hold.

Cross-Cradle

With this position, you start with baby's weight on your arm. You want to be able to move their body across you and if you're just holding their head, it may feel like you're yanking them uncomfortably. The whole baby moves when we do 'baby to breast'. You support their head by holding them round the ears, neck and top of their back. Imagine Elvis at the end of his career is Las Vegas. Your hand is the big Elvis collar. You want to check there isn't clothing bunched up between you. A bra rolled down with a breast pad squashed inside it could push baby's chest far away enough from your body that it affects the way baby will attach. Baby's hands also can't be between you. The bottom arm can be hugging your body and round towards your armpit or right down their side by their hip. Lots of new mums say that the baby's hands are 'getting in the way' and it can seem to be very frustrating. Remember that baby uses its hands to help it find the breast and centre itself. If you can get

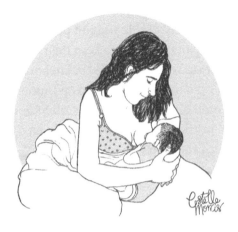

baby's chin and face to the breast quickly, you'll find that very often the arms will instantly calm. Dab the baby's nose against the nipple and wait for the gape.

Take a moment. It's OK for this bit to take a couple of minutes at least. They will hopefully gape and tilt their head as they reach up for the nipple. When you feel you've got that gape, you're going to move baby's body quickly and plonk them on. Their bottom lip will be as far away from the nipple as possible. Just check your arm is well-supported. You're not going to be able to hold the weight of a baby's head throughout a feed on just a few fingers. It's often a good idea to bring your other arm round and support baby's head on that forearm. So start in a cross-cradle hold and then move into a cradle hold. You might even be then able to move your cross-cradle arm out slowly and leave baby in a cradle position. That gives you a spare hand for essentials like drinking, eating and reading.

Or you might have cushions supporting your cross-cradle arm and taking baby's weight. Another option is that you lean back so that baby's weight is going through your torso. What's going to be hard is an increasingly heavy baby balancing on your arms and hands as you sit bolt upright. By the way, you don't need to sit upright for the milk to flow. The milk will flow even if you are leaning right back. It's your milk ejection reflex, the baby creating negative space in their mouth and the baby's tongue that moves the milk around. Gravity doesn't have a lot to do with it.

One thing worth remembering, some women have naturally shorter forearms. You may not be able to have baby resting on your arm and be able to support the base of their head. Your arm may literally not be long enough. So if this position seems to be a struggle, you're not going mad. You just needed a few more centimetres of arm. You may do better with a bit of cradle hold and using both arms for support, the rugby hold or a more laid-back position, or let baby's bottom slip off your arm slightly.

Cradle-hold

This is often the picture we imagine when we visualise breastfeeding for the first time. Unfortunately there aren't many images of the Mother Mary and baby Jesus doing the rugby hold or laid-back breastfeeding. Baby's head is resting somewhere around the crook of your elbow. Their body is close to yours and their hands aren't squished between you. No clothing bunched between

*The baby's nose may sometimes
be touching your breast. This is
particularly likely if you have
larger softer breasts.*

you. You dab baby's nose around the nipple and when they gape, you bring them even closer to your body. You want their chin massaging the breast. Their head is ideally slightly tilted which gives them even more chance that the chin and tongue have good breast contact. When you bring them nice and close with that gape, focus on two things. First, you want their bottom lip to come as far away from the nipple as possible. It's OK if the top lip is much closer. If you see any areola (and there's going to be a lot of variation with this as areolas come in lots of different sizes), you can see some areola above the top lip but none below the chin. Secondly, try and picture the nipple heading up towards the roof of their mouth. You're aiming for a point on the roof of their mouth rather than heading down towards the back of their throat. Once baby is on, check that you are well-supported. If you had to lean forward and move the breast around, something is probably going to adjust during the feed in a way we don't want it to. Baby will have moved to you. Baby to breast is the phrase we say. We want you to finish a feed

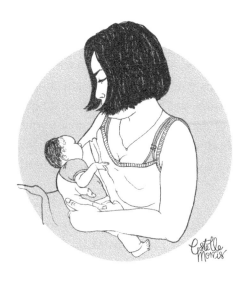

as comfortably as when you started. You shouldn't have back ache or feel relief that your arm no longer has to do any work. If you finish a feed rubbing your sore arm or hand and thinking, "'Glad that's over it," something needs to change. You may have been slightly slipping during a feed without even realising it if something was uncomfortable. We only have to move a few millimetres for problems to start. The baby's nose may sometimes be touching your breast. This is particularly likely if you have larger softer breasts. It's not panic stations if a baby's nose does make contact, as babies will prioritise breathing and come off and adjust if they need to. You can tuck their bottom in a bit more and see if that tilts them so that their nose is a little more free. Ideally you'll have got them on anyway with that head tilt that drives their chin in without burying the nose into the breast. What we want to avoid is pressing a finger into the breast to keep breast tissue away from the nose. That's not a great plan for various reasons. Firstly it means you are potentially affecting the flow of milk by pressing on a milk duct –some are quite close to the surface of the skin. It can also increase your chance of getting milk ducts and possibly mastitis. It's also taking the emphasis away from that good quality head tilt.

Lying down

Being able to breastfeed while lying down is one of the essential breastfeeding mummy skills. It's right up there with being able to eat one-handed and opening a clasp on a nursing bra without losing your marbles. You might think you can get up all through the night and breastfeed in a chair but after a few weeks of that, it starts to become considerably less fun. When you breastfeed lying down you can rest and you may even be able to sleep. 70-80% of breastfeeding families have the baby sleeping in their bed with them at some point. It's a really good idea to read more about bed-sharing and some of the risk factors so you can understand how to do it as safely as possible. I recommend visiting ISIS online: https://www.isisonline. org.uk/where_babies_sleep/parents_bed/. The Infant Sleep Information Source is an excellent resource filled with useful accessible evidence-based information. It's the place to visit if you want information about safe sleep for your baby.

When you breastfeed lying down, the principles of

good attachment are the same. We still want that nice wide gape. We still want baby's body close to mum's body. What often works well is to have both mum and baby on their side. Take a moment to look at the bedding around you. Ideally your duvet is tucked under you or well away so it can't flop on to baby. You may be determined that you won't fall asleep while you are feeding but it's sensible to think through what might happen if you did. Make sure baby is far away from your pillow. Perhaps put your pillow on a diagonal away from him. What is on the other side of baby? Babies can move surprisingly far even when they are very small. They can get trapped between walls and beds. Partners that aren't breastfeeding don't benefit from hormones that keep you more tuned into baby so it isn't recommended to have baby in the middle between you.

One option is to have a side-car cot next to your bed and that's behind baby when she feeds. After the feed, you may be able to slide her back into her space but if not, at least if she did move, she's only got her cot space behind her. Read the guidelines carefully when you set up your cot. Some mums are so worried about falling asleep with baby in the bed that they get up and move to a sofa. It is far more dangerous to fall asleep on a chair or sofa than it is in a bed when you are following the safety guidelines.

When it's time for latching, have your baby's nose level with your nipple. Nose to nipple is particularly important in this position. We really want baby to be reaching up and tilting their head back to get to the breast. This will give their tongue optimum space on the breast, really get the chin pressing in nicely and help their nose to be as clear as possible (though some mums with larger softer breasts may still find baby's nose touches). When the baby tilts and you get that gape, you press in on the top of their back and bring them as close as possible. You'll probably need to keep that hand there so their chin and body stays close. If you do fall asleep, your hand may start to relax and the baby may end up rolling onto their back to sleep once the feed has finished. When it's time for the other breast, switch yourself round so your head is at the other end of the bed. Go 'top to tail'. Your breasts will be again on the outside and baby will be in the safer outside position in the bed (assuming there's a partner on the other side).

Pick the position that seems to work best for your baby, your breasts, your chair, your life. If you can have a couple up your sleeve that's useful because it means the breast will get drained in different ways and it gives

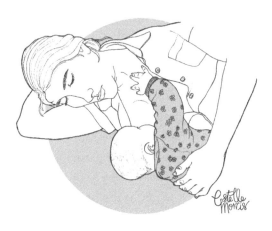

you options depending on where you are. Most mums do appreciate the opportunity to lie down so being able to breastfeed in bed is certainly worth practising. Quite often people are loyal to the position that works best for them but there any many different options – including several not described here. If you are comfortable and baby can get the milk out effectively and you can reach the remote control – those are the things that really matter.

How to Train as a Breastfeeding Counsellor

Do you think you might want to train as a breastfeeding counsellor?

Here's a quick quiz...

1. Do you find a woman breastfeeding in public puts you off your coffee because...
   (a) It's a bit awkward, or
   (b) You sit there wondering whether she'd mind if you went up to her and congratulated her for feeding in a café (and after much deliberation you eventually decide on the 'warm smile/ thumbs up' combo).

If you answered 'a', this is probably not the chapter for you.

2. Can your facebook wall easily display photos of the breasts of five different women from two different continents in one week?
3. Does your partner mention to pregnant strangers that

they might want to talk to you about breastfeeding?

4. Does your mum save newspaper clippings of articles on breastfeeding? (When you actually heard about the article two weeks ago and have already have three online discussions about it).

5. Do you wish everyone could breastfeed for as long as they want to and you get frustrated when you hear that doesn't always happen?

This may be for you then.

Becoming a breastfeeding counsellor in the UK is fundamentally about volunteering your time to help mothers to reach their own breastfeeding goals. You will need to be able to empathise, offer emotional support and information. You will need to appreciate that not all breastfeeding mothers look the same or make the same choices. You will not be offering 'advice' but empowering mums (and their partners) to make their own decisions.

It is immensely important and rewarding work and breastfeeding counsellors are desperately needed.

It's worth noting that this is not going to be a new career path for most people who train as a breastfeeding counsellor. If you train as an NCT practitioner, you may be able to make a career out of it. There are also some paid breastfeeding support roles available in some parts of the country depending on projects in your area, but these are few and far between. What is for sure is that the skills you learn, the experiences you have, the people you meet will make this worthwhile – both in a 'future employment' sense and a wider 'life-changing' sense.

There are four main organisations you can train with in the UK. There are som e things different about the training (cost, location, philosophy of the organisations).

There are some things that are the same about all of them:

- You'll be focusing on the needs of the mother and baby and putting your personal experiences to one side whenever possible.
- You will use good listening skills to support mums and their families.
- You will be expected to provide evidence-based information. That means information based on science, research and best practice. You won't be giving personal opinions.
- You'll be working as a team with other people supporting the mum. You may refer to GPs or health visitors or midwives. Breastfeeding counsellors don't work in isolation and are great at sign-posting to other services.
- You'll get on-going training and supervision to help you in your role.

Here's how you can go about getting trained:

If you want to train with the NCT, you have a couple of options. You can take the paid option to become a self-employed NCT practitioner. http://www.nct.org.uk/nct-college/work-opportunities#level5 NCT BFCs may take sessions of antenatal classes, run support groups and work on the NCT helpline. The course costs approximately £7000 and takes two years to complete. It can be done in less time if you study full-time. There are some bursaries available. You study for a foundation degree with the University of Worcester and take the 'breastfeeding pathway'. You start with the essentials course to become a 'birth and beyond practitioner' and then go onto do the breastfeeding specialism. You will need to have breastfed one child for at least six months. The breastfeeding pathway consists of three modules (counselling skills, applying counselling skills, understanding women's experiences of breastfeeding): each requiring two study days and five tutorials. Some of the study days will be at the University of Worcester and some arranged in a more local area depending on numbers of students. The course will include writing a 3000 word essay, short answer questions, tutor group discussions and a range of learning experiences.

If you train with La Leche League, you'll be called a La Leche League leader rather than a breastfeeding counsellor: https://www.laleche.org.uk/content/thinking-about-lll-leadership.

It's a good idea to read the La Leche League book, 'The Womanly Art of Breastfeeding' (which is a good read for anyone interested in breastfeeding) and familiarise yourself with the ten concepts that are important to La Leche League. That's not to say a La Leche League leader wouldn't support any breastfeeding mother whatever her parenting views but just that the La Leche League is underpinned by a philosophy that will shape your appreciation of the mother/ child relationship and all leaders will share: https://www. laleche.org.uk/sites/default/files/LAD%20Brochure%20 final%20Jan%202011.pdf

You should also find out if there are La Leche League meetings local to you and attend some

https://www.laleche.org.uk/find-lll-group

You'll be expected to have breastfed for at least nine months. Many leaders train with an established leader at an established meeting but if you don't have one close enough to you, there are other ways of doing it. The training is a combination of face-to-face and written work and can take two years depending on your pace. The pace will be very individual to you and might depend on things like the age of your children. You can find out the current fees by contacting LLLGB.

La Leche League leaders will usually support at a local meeting (they may share running a meeting with other leaders) and can also support on the LLL helpline.

You can also become a breastfeeding supporter with the Breastfeeding Network. That's their word for a breastfeeding counsellor equivalent – not to be confused with 'peer supporters' from other organisations who will have done a shorter course. Training happens locally and is face-to-face: http://www.breastfeedingnetwork.org.uk/ get-involved/train-to-be-a-registered-volunteer/

Opportunities depend on funding and what is available in your local area. This is what is currently available: http:// www.breastfeedingnetwork.org.uk/get-involved/train-to-be-a-registered-volunteer/areas-where-we-are-able-to-provide-some-training/

You will not have to pay any training fees. You start by training as a breastfeeding HELPER and then you can go on to do the supporter training if it's available. Helper training consists of twelve two-hour sessions and babes-in-arms are welcome. Supporter training usually takes approximately two years to complete. The expectation is you will volunteer for the BfN after your training by offering face-to-face support at groups or on the BfN helpline or National Breastfeeding Helpline (phone or web chat). The training will often take place in tutors' homes and consists of written and oral work.

The last charity you can train with is the Association of Breastfeeding Mothers. Like the Breastfeeding Network, you start with the first level course (which the ABM calls 'Mother Supporter' course) and then you can go on to train to become a breastfeeding counsellor which takes approximately eighteen months to two years. http://abm.me.uk/about-the-abm/training-with-the-association-of-breastfeeding-mothers/

You need to have breastfed for a minimum of six months before you apply. The course costs £100 and you also have to be a member of the ABM. It is then expected that counsellors volunteer on the helpline for a minimum of two years after training. The ABM helps run the National Breastfeeding Helpline with the BfN and have their own helpline. Many ABM counsellors also support in their local community. The ABM training is a distance learning programme. This means that you submit written modules and communicate with tutors via email and phone and through online discussion. There are some practical activities such as observations and practice phone calls and you are required to attend one study day a year. The advantage of a home study course is that you don't have to leave young children and the training can happen anywhere. However it is not a learning style that works for everyone and requires independent organisation and reading at home. There are eight additional modules after the initial Mother Supporter course has been completed.

So those are your options. If you read those descriptions and felt excitement and anticipation, this may be a path for you. If you read them and thought, "that sounds like a tremendous hassle" – perhaps not.

There are other ways you can support mothers depending on your passion and your experience:

- You may be interested in becoming a doula (breastfeeding support is often part of a doula's role too): http://doula.org.uk/content/becoming-doula
- Or perhaps training to become a home start volunteer: http://www.home-start.org.uk/volunteer/
- Or volunteering for a charity like Bliss: http://www.bliss.org.uk/get-involved/ or PANDAS, who help mums with depression:
- http://www.pandasfoundation.org.uk/get-involved/volunteering.html#.VHSVZYusXg8

On Twitter and Facebook, you'll find counsellors and trainers from all of these organisations who I'm sure will be happy to answer any of your questions.

If you have the time and the inclination, you can make an incredible difference to the lives of new mums and babies. Your commitment is desperately needed.

Check websites for current updates.

If Breastfeeding Doesn't Work Out...

If you end up not breastfeeding, it may be that exclusive pumping is an option for you. That means bottle-feeding with only breastmilk in the bottle. Exclusive pumping was hard to achieve even just a few years ago but now modern electric breast pumps make it a real possibility for many mums. I recommend you get hold of a book called 'Exclusively pumping Breast milk' by Stephanie Casemore. It's a great guide to the practicalities, and pretty much everything else, of this subject. It can be incredibly hard work but also immensely rewarding.

Whatever ends up being in the bottle, it's really important to know that bottle feeding can happen in a way that is more likely to maximise the opportunities for bonding and emotional nurturing. You can bottle feed skin-to-skin. Yes, you can. Just because you don't see people doing it on telly or in Starbucks it doesn't mean it can't be what you do every day at home. You can also feed in response to your baby's feeding cues rather than to the clock. You may want to use a technique called Paced Bottle-feeding (have a look on YouTube) to check that the flow stays as slow as possible and baby uses their tongue and jaw muscles to create negative space and more some work. This may help in preventing them from overfeeding.

You should also swap sides just like breastfeeders do. This means that visual development is more likely to be the norm. Imagine if you always bottle-feed on the same side – how might that affect the development of the eye and associated neurological development on the constantly blinkered side?

You may want to investigate the world of donor milk using an informal milk-banking site like HM4MB (human milk for human babies) and Eats for Feets. There are facebook groups with families seeking milk donors and mothers offering their milk. A typical post might say: "Hi, I'm in Oxfordshire and I have 30oz in my freezer to go to a good home. Non-smoker. Can deliver locally." It is possible to pasteurise donor milk in your home to reduce the risk of infection.

Just a word on formula types, you may feel like goat's milk or soya milk is more 'natural' but we don't have evidence to support this. Soya formula means exposing babies to high levels of hormones called phytoestrogens. The NHS site states that 'it is likely that they could affect babies' reproductive development'. If you want to learn a bit more about formula types then the charity First Steps Nutrition Trust has some useful resources (firststepsnutrition.org). The bottom line is that there is not much difference between the major brands of formula. It is fine to stay on a first formula until a baby is twelve

*Every day you managed to breastfeed
counts. Every feed counted.*

months old and there's no need to switch to follow-on milk. At twelve months, you can then start using full-fat cow's milk.

Please know that breastfeeding does not have to be 'all or nothing'. A mum who pumps just once a day and bottle-feeds 30mls of breastmilk is doing something immensely worthwhile, giving their baby tailor-made 'medicine' with huge immunological benefits. Perhaps you can breastfeed once or twice a day. A mum who doesn't seem to make enough milk does not have to give up breastfeeding. Any breastmilk is beneficial.

Perhaps you can return to breastfeeding after a break. You can absolutely restart breastfeeding and relactate even after a break of several weeks or months. A breastfeeding counsellor or lactation consultant can talk you through how to do this. The ABM have also produced a useful leaflet: http://abm.me.uk/restarting-breastfeeding-after-a-gap/

That was all the practical stuff. I know the idea of not breastfeeding can sometimes be immensely painful and difficult. Sometimes we are very concerned that new mums shouldn't feel 'guilty' when in fact it is also important to acknowledge that mourning the loss of breastfeeding is something that mothers are allowed to do and these emotions are perfectly valid.

We all make decisions based on our circumstances and the opportunities available to us. Not everyone can access top-quality breastfeeding support. Not everyone has support from their family and friends. A small minority of mums may physically struggle to produce a full milk supply. If breastfeeding is too difficult for you and you feel you need to move on, be kind to yourself. That's what you needed to do. It was something that felt right based on what was best for your family and you. It's my personal experience that mothers who take their time to consider the decision carefully and talk to people along the way, can move on without regrets. Every day you managed to breastfeed counts. Every feed counted.

Please know that breastfeeding does not have to be 'all or nothing'. A mum who pumps just once a day and bottle feeds 30mls of breastmilk is doing something immensely worthwhile

More Reading

Websites

There are lots of websites out there about breastfeeding and motherhood. Some are blogs and mums sharing their personal experiences which can be supportive, meaningful and touching. Others are information-based resources written by professionals and trained experts. Whenever you absorb a piece of information, just check where it came from. The internet is your great mate and your not-so-great mate when it comes to accurate information on breastfeeding. It's also worth remembering that some information is paid for by the baby food and baby milk industry. They may sometimes have their logos at the top of the page but they can also call themselves different things and work in subtle ways. Their information may talk about how breastfeeding mums need to be really careful to eat healthily or emphasise sore nipples even in a jokey and apparently harmless way. Or put a huge emphasis on the necessity of pumping and using bottles to make breastfeeding manageable.

I would recommend: **www.kellymom.com**

As I often say, not the best name in the world for an evidence-based reliable website run by a respected lactation consultant but it is a site that is extremely comprehensive and bases its information on research and good sources. They have a discussion forum too.

I would also recommend **breastfeeding.support**. This is a site created by UK IBCLC Philippa Pearson-Glaze. It has an excellent range of articles and is growing as a respected resource for parents and professionals.

The charities run by the main breastfeeding charities will also be reliable. As mentioned before, the Breastfeeding Network is particularly strong on medication and combining medical procedures with breastfeeding. **www.breastfeedingnetwork.org.uk**

There's also some really valuable information here: **http://www.unicef.org.uk/BabyFriendly/News-and-Research/Research/Breastfeeding-research---An-overview/**

If you want to rent a hospital grade breast pump, your local NCT pump agent may be a good place to start and your local NCT branch should have their details: **http://www.nct.org.uk/branches**

You can also rent breast pumps from **www.ardobreastpumps.co.uk**

Dr. Jack Newman is a name you'll hear a lot in the world of breastfeeding support. His website has some really useful videos that give you a sense of newborn latching, particularly important if you haven't seen much breastfeeding up close before. His breast compressions technique can also be really useful to encourage a baby to drink more at the breast, perhaps if they are excessively sleepy. **http://www.breastfeedinginc.ca/index.php**

Association of Breastfeeding Mothers (**www.abm. me.uk**) for leaflets and information on a range of topics such as restarting breastfeeding after a gap, antenatal expression of colostrum, reflux and ways that dads and grandparents can support during breastfeeding.

If your baby is unwell or if you are spending time in hospital, I urge you to read **http://www.heartmummy. co.uk/**. There is still a common misconception that unwell babies will be 'tired out' by breastfeeding based on a lack of understanding of the mechanics of breastfeeding. We know much more than we once did with modern ultrasound research. We also know more about the stresses bottle-feeding can bring in comparison to breastfeeding. If your baby is unable to breastfeed, it's important their carers know why it's even more important that they receive breast milk.

If you want to find out more about doulas, visit **www. doula.org.uk**. They can support new mums in pregnancy and birth but also beyond to help get breastfeeding established and manage daily life in the first few weeks.

The internet is your great mate and your not-so-great mate when it comes to accurate information on breastfeeding.

Twitter is also an easy place to find breastfeeding experts and mums who know where to find you help. Use the hashtag #breastfeeding. Look for me (@makesmilk) and I'll try and point you in the right direction.

On Facebook, look for **Dispelling Breastfeeding Myths.** Look for local groups to find nearby mums. Look for pages and groups connected to the breastfeeding charities.

Books

Here is a list of many of the books a typical lactation consultant will have on her shelves. There are other books on our shelves that we'd rather others didn't read (so we might hide those in Waterstones).

The Womanly Art of Breastfeeding **by La Leche League International**

The Food of Love: your formula for successful breastfeeding **by Kate Evans**

The Breastfeeding Mother's Guide to Making More Milk **by Diana West and Lisa Marasco**

Breastfeeding without birthing by Alyssa Schnell

Breastfeeding, Take Two by Stephanie Casemore

Breastfeeding Older Children by Ann Sinnott

The Politics of Breastfeeding **by Gabrielle Palmer**

Breastfeeding: stories to inspire and inform edited by Susan Last

Bestfeeding by Mary Renfrew, Chloe Fisher, Suzanne Arms

The Breastfeeding Atlas by Barbara Wilson-Clay

The Breastfeeding Cafe: Mothers Share the Joys, Challenges, and Secrets of Nursing by Barbara L. Behrmann

Fresh Milk by Fiona Giles

Breastfeeding and Human Lactation by Karen Wambach and Jan Riordan

Core Curriculum for Lactation Consultant Practice ILCA

Dr. Jack Newman's Guide to Breastfeeding by Newman, Jack, Dr. and Teresa Pitman

Ina May's Guide to Breastfeeding by Ina May Gaskin

***Supporting Sucking Skills In Breastfeeding Infants* by Catherine Watson Genna**

Medications & Mothers' Milk by Thomas W. Hale and Hilary E. Rowe

So That's What They're For! The Definitive Breastfeeding Guide by Janet Tamaro

The Breastfeeding Answer Book by Nancy Mohrbacher and Julie Stock (though getting older now and you'll need to find the update available online)

Defining your Own Success: Breastfeeding After Breast Reduction Surgery by Diana West

Adventures in Tandem Nursing: Breastfeeding During Pregnancy and Beyond by Hilary Flower

Baby-Led breastfeeding by Gill Rapley and Tracey Murkett

Exclusively pumping breast milk by Stephanie Casemore

<u>*Mothering and Parenting*</u>

What Mother's Do, especially when it looks like nothing by
    Naomi Stadlen

Why love matters: how affection shapes a baby's brain by Sue
    Gerhardt.

The Baby book by Dr William Sears

Why Doulas matter by Maddie McMahon

<u>*Sleep*</u>

*Sweet Sleep: Night-time and Naptime Strategies for the
    Breastfeeding Family* by La Leche League International
    (Diane Wiessinger and Diana West)

*The No-Cry Sleep Solution: Gentle Ways to Help Your Baby
    Sleep Through the Night* by Elizabeth Pantley

The No-Cry Sleep solution for toddlers and pre-schoolers by
    Elizabeth Pantley

<u>*Starting Solids*</u>

***Baby-Led weaning: Helping your baby to love good food* by
    Gill Rapley and Tracey Murkett**

The Baby-Led weaning cookbook by Gill Rapley and Tracey
    Murkett

Index